Nephrology Nursing Scope and Standards of Practice

8th Edition

Editor
Norma J. Gomez, MBA, MSN, RN, CNNe

American Nephrology Nurses Association
www.annanurse.org

Nephrology Nursing Scope and Standards of Practice
8th Edition

ISBN 978-1-940325-32-3

Editor
Norma J. Gomez

Publication Management
Anthony J. Jannetti, Inc.
East Holly Avenue/Box 56, Pitman, New Jersey 08071-0056

Managing Editor: Claudia Cuddy
Editorial Assistant: Joseph Tonzelli
Layout Design and Production: Claudia Cuddy
Cover Design: Darin Peters
Design Consultant: Jack M. Bryant
Executive Director: Mike Cunningham

ANNA Disclaimer
The *Nephrology Nursing Scope and Standards of Practice* is designed to provide information and assist decision making. If a clinician is looking for prescriptive information regarding the management of the patient with kidney disease, he or she should examine literature with the most current evidence-based information.

American Nephrology Nurses Association
East Holly Avenue/Box 56, Pitman, New Jersey 08071-0056
www.annanurse.org ▪ Email: anna@annanurse.org ▪ Phone: 888-600-2662

Contents

Approval and Acknowledgment by American Nurses Association

The American Nurses Association has approved the Nephrology Nursing Scope of Practice as defined herein.

The American Nurses Association has acknowledged the Nephrology Nursing Standards of Practice as set forth herein.

October 19, 2016

Foreword

ANNA's *Nephrology Nursing Scope and Standards of Practice* are a set of guidelines to guide evidence-based practice and delivery of high-quality nursing care. Since the first edition of the standards was published in 1977, there have been many changes in nephrology care, and new evidence is available. This is the eighth edition. This edition incorporates the newest evidence and changes in practice. It should serve as a basis for clinical quality and, when necessary, as a resource for legal issues when they arise regarding quality of care.

Norma Gomez, MBA, MSN, RN, CNNe, has served as Project Director and Editor for the last two editions of the ANNA *Nephrology Nursing Scope and Standards of Practice*. The ANNA Board of Directors and I would like to thank and commend Norma and each of the contributors to this edition for their time and valuable input.

We hope that you will use this edition as you continue to provide quality care to our patients

Sheila Doss-McQuitty, MBA, BSN, RN, CNN, CCRA
ANNA President, 2016–2017

Preface

The recently revised *American Nurses Association's (ANA) Nursing: Scope and Standards of Practice* (2015) provides both a broad foundation for defining nursing practice and a comprehensive guide for the evaluation of that practice. There was an additional standard added related to culturally congruent practice as well as defined competencies for the graduate-level prepared nurse.

The American Nephrology Nurses Association (ANNA) *Nephrology Nursing Scope and Standards of Practice, 8th Edition,* has been revised and updated for nephrology nursing and presents a similar approach as the ANA standards. An editor and workgroup were identified to revise the current nephrology nursing scope and standards of practice. The workgroup developed a project plan and contacted experts in the field. The Specialty Practice Networks (SPNs) were involved in the review process. Draft revisions were posted on the ANNA website for member response.

The 8th edition of the ANNA standards provides an updated definition of nephrology nursing and scope of practice statement. The section of examples on how to use the standards in clinical practice presents a short vignette with an overview of a situation that requires intervention by the nephrology nurse. Samples of tools that incorporate the standards into the various situations are included.

A glossary has been included to aid with the understanding of terms used in all the sections. Examples of the terms used in this edition include *kidney replacement therapies (KRT)* in place of *renal replacement therapies (RRT)* and *healthcare consumer* used synonymously with *patient*. The term *family* relates to family of origin or significant others as identified by the patient.

In brief, the *Nephrology Nursing Scope and Standards of Practice* provides nephrology nursing with a method of defining the scope of its practice and a conduit for the evaluation of that practice. Moreover, this document serves as a guide in the identification of nephrology nurses' responsibilities to their profession, their colleagues, and the healthcare consumer.

Norma J. Gomez, MBA, MSN, RN, CNNe
Editor

Acknowledgments

Sincere appreciation is extended to the ANNA Board of Directors for their commitment to quality patient care.

Special acknowledgment goes to the editors, contributors, and reviewers of previous editions of ANNA's Standards of Clinical Practice:

1977	*Standards of Clinical Practice for the Nephrology Patient*
1982	*Nephrology Nursing Standards of Clinical Practice*
1988	*ANNA Standards of Clinical Practice for Nephrology Nursing*
1993	*Standards of Clinical Practice for Nephrology Nursing*
1999	*Standards and Guidelines of Clinical Practice for Nephrology Nursing*
2005	*Nephrology Nursing Standards of Practice and Guidelines for Care*
2011	*Nephrology Nursing Scope and Standards of Practice*

Thank you to Beth Ulrich and Caroline Counts for their work on the ANA application for specialty practice recognition.

Special appreciation goes to Claudia Cuddy, Managing Editor, for her help in making this edition a reality.

Contributors and Reviewers

Contributors

Norma J. Gomez, MBA, MSN, RN, CNNe
Safety and Infection Prevention Program Manager
Satellite Healthcare
San Jose, California

Debra Castner, APN, RN, CNN
Nurse Practitioner
Jersey Coast Nephrology and Hypertension Associates
Brick, New Jersey

Debra J Hain, PhD, ARNP, ANP-BC, GNP-BC, FAANP, FNKF
Associate Professor/Lead AGNP Faculty, Tenured
Florida Atlantic University
Christine E Lynn College of Nursing
Boca Raton, Florida

Reviewers

Virginia Abeyta, DNP
Nephrology RN
Puget Sound Veterans Hospital, Seattle, WA

Karen Joann Gaietto, MSN, BSN, RN, CNN
Acute Clinical Service Specialist
Davita Healthcare Partners Inc., Tiffin, OH

Mary Hannan, MSN, APN, AGACNP-BC
Associate Dean of Faculty
Chamberlain College of Nursing

Reviewers continue on next page

Carolyn E. Latham, DNP, MSN, MBA, CNN, RN
Consultant
Nashville, TN

Maryam Lyon, MSN, RN, CNN
Nursing Professor
Hondros College, Fairborn, OH

Molly Mickle, BSN, RN, CNN
Regional Home Therapies Manager
Fresenius, Niskayuna, NY

Cynthia J. Oliveri, RN, CDN
Education Coordinator
Fresenius Kidney Care
Colonia, NJ

Maria O'Shaughnessy, MSN, RN, CNN, CNL
Adjunct Faculty/Home Therapies Nurse
University of San Francisco/Satellite Healthcare–WellBound
San Francisco/San Jose, CA

Jennifer Payton, MHCA, BSN, RN, CNN
Clinical Support Specialist
HealthStar CES, Mahwah, NJ

Sherry Rivera, DNP, APRN, ANP-C
Nurse Practitioner
New Orleans Nephrology Associates, Marrero, LA

Section 1 Nephrology Nursing Scope of Practice

Definition of Nephrology Nursing

Nephrology nursing is a specialty practice addressing the protection, promotion, and optimization of health abilities, prevention of illness and injury, facilitation of healing, alleviation of suffering through the diagnosis and treatment of human response, and advocacy in the care of individuals, families, groups, communities, and populations affected by kidney disease.

Scope of Practice for Nephrology Nursing

The scope of practice for nephrology nursing describes, for the public and the profession, the nature of this specialty's nursing practice. The specialty's scope is derived from the scope of nursing practice as defined by the American Nurses Association (ANA) (2015) and builds on the previous versions published by the American Nephrology Nurses Association (ANNA).

Nephrology nursing encompasses the primary, secondary, and tertiary care of individuals with potential and progressive chronic kidney disease (CKD), end-stage renal disease (ESRD), acute kidney injury (AKI), and other healthcare conditions requiring nephrologic intervention. Nephrology nursing practice spans the continuum of care for patients with kidney disease. Nephrology nurses provide care to neonatal, pediatric, adult, and older adults in all racial/ethnic groups. The nursing care can be complex, as these patient populations may have various comorbid conditions, including cardiovascular disease, diabetes, hypertension, infectious disease, and/or mineral and bone disease. In addition, many face psychosocial issues, such as depression and anxiety.

To provide clearer understanding, the term *kidney replacement therapies (KRT)* is now being used in the nephrology community in place of the term *renal replacement therapies (RRT)*. These terms identify all therapies used to treat kidney disease, including dialysis, transplantation, and palliative care. Throughout this publication, the terms *healthcare consumer* and *patient* will be used interchangeably. *Healthcare consumer* is defined as the patient, person, client, family, group, community, or population who is the focus of attention and to whom the registered nurse is providing services as sanctioned by the state regulatory bodies (ANA, 2015b). The term *family* relates to the family of origin or significant others as identified by the patient.

The ANNA work group authoring this edition determined to continue the usage of *interdisciplinary* as reflected in the Centers for Medicare and Medicaid Services (CMS) Conditions for Coverage (CfCs) (CMS, 2008), rather than move to the more contemporary term, *interprofessional*. The interdisciplinary team is composed of a diverse group of healthcare professionals. The members are recognized for their expertise and individual roles. Issues may be referred for collaboration to professionals within or outside one's own profession as warranted. Interdisciplinary collaboration within the nephrology community may impact professional practice boundaries in the effort to improve the health of the population living with kidney disease, reduce healthcare costs, and enhance the quality of healthcare delivery.

Overview of the Scope of Practice for Nephrology Nursing

The recognition of kidney disease, acute and chronic, as a major health problem has led to the development of nephrology nursing as a specialty. The practice of nephrology nursing encompasses the roles of direct caregiver, educator, coordinator, consultant, administrator, and researcher. The practice extends to all care delivery settings in which patients are at risk for developing or are experiencing chronic kidney disease (CKD) stages 1 through 5, and receive health care, education, and counseling for kidney disease prevention, diagnosis, progression, and treatment.

Optimal individual physical and cognitive function and family support throughout all phases of disease management are the primary goals of nephrology nursing. The nephrology nurse achieves these primary goals by diagnosing and treating human responses exhibited by individuals and families with kidney disease or who are at risk for developing CKD. These human responses include, but are not limited to, physical symptoms, functional limitations, psychosocial disruptions, and knowledge needs.

Treatment of these responses involves health promotion and disease prevention counseling, health maintenance education, psychosocial support to build or sustain coping capacity, education to encourage active participation in decision making and self-care, restorative physical care to manage disease and treatment-related symptoms, and the delivery of kidney-replacement therapies, including transplantation.

The focus of the nephrology nurse is the patient, an entity that can include individuals, families, groups, and communities. Nephrology nurses manage care to meet the individualized needs of the patient with kidney disease to maximize independence and quality of life.

Nephrology nursing practice occurs throughout the patient's life span, along a continuum of care and across delivery settings. Care requirements extend beyond kidney disease to address acute and/or chronic causative disease processes, as well as subsequent comorbid complications. The nature of this nursing care spans the spectrum from preventive and acute through replacement therapies and rehabilitation, as well as palliative, supportive care. Nephrology nursing may be provided in a variety of settings that include, but are not limited to, inpatient, outpatient, freestanding clinics, and home care.

All nephrology nurses are legally, ethically, and morally responsible for practicing in accordance with recognized standards of professional nursing practice and professional performance, the recognized professional code of ethics, and specialty certification.

The Model of Professional Nursing Practice Regulation (2015) illustrates the scope and standards and provides the foundation for our practice (ANA, 2015). The apex of the model of professional responsibility is achieved with the individual nephrology nurse's assumption of personal accountability for continuing education and professional experience over and above the basic requirements.

Integrating the Art and Science of Nursing

General Nephrology Nursing Practice

This section provides an overview of nephrology nursing practice within the profession of nursing. Nursing as a profession is defined as both a science and an art that generates new knowledge from nursing research and other disciplines and applies the best available evidence to inform clinical practice. Nursing research is a process of scientific discovery guided by a theoretical framework.

The nephrology nurse coordinates care in collaboration with other care providers and health team members to plan and provide required care as effectively and safely as possible. The nephrology nurse acts as a patient guide and advocate, assisting the patient in seeking information, assuring that the patient has the opportunity for informed consent for treatment decisions, and promoting the maximal level of patient-desired independence. The nephrology nurse may also function in the role as a nurse manager to assure patient safety and the delivery of appropriate care.

The nephrology nurse is accountable for delivering care within the framework of the nursing process. The nephrology nurse uses assessment findings to formulate nursing diagnoses and prioritize problems according to patient need and preference. The nephrology nurse engages the patient in mutual goal setting and collaboration in developing a plan of care directed toward achieving identified goals. The effectiveness of the plan of care in goal achievement is evaluated through patient outcomes.

The nephrology nurse actively participates in professional role development activities including continuing education, quality assessment and improvement, and the review and clinical application of research findings to assure evidence-based practice. The nephrology nurse develops ethically sound practice and confronts ethical challenges through application of the *Nephrology Nursing Scope and Standards of Practice.*

Theoretical Foundations of Nursing

To advance nursing science and practice, it is essential that nephrology nurses caring for individuals with chronic kidney disease across the healthcare continuum understand the essence of a metaparadigm of nursing. Theory is a way of viewing a phenomenon that is of concern within the discipline (Smith, 2014). The metaparadigm of nursing is "a framework for the discipline that sets forth the phenomena of interest and the propositions, principles, and methods of the discipline" (Parker, 2005, p. 5). The metaparadigm provides a conceptual context to develop and test conceptual models and nursing theories. Historically a metaparadigm of nursing describes the concepts of person, environment, health, and nursing. A relatively new metaparadigm of nursing includes concepts that support four domains: (1) client, (2) client-nurse encounters, (3) practice, and (4) environment (Kim, 1987).

Nursing focuses on the promotion and maintenance of health and the prevention or resolution of disease, illness, or disability. The nursing needs of human beings are identified from a holistic perspective and are met within the context of a culturally sensitive, caring interpersonal relationship (ANA, 2010b). Conceptual and theoretical frameworks provide the foundation for nursing research and evidence-based practice to advance the discipline of nursing. "The discipline of nursing is formed by a community of scholars, including nurses in all venues, who share a commitment to values, knowledge, and processes to guide thought and work of the discipline" (Smith & Parker, 2013, p. 4). On the ladder of abstraction, the metaparadigm is at the top, followed by grand theories, then middle-range theories and finally, research and practice traditions that are related to grand and middle-range theories (Smith, 2014). Nephrology nursing practice encompasses protocols and guidelines that emerge from these theories.

Science is concerned with relationship and causality (cause and effect). The scientific approach to understanding a phenomenon includes observation, verifiability, and experience, hypothesis testing, and experimentation, which is part of the scientific method. In a dynamic healthcare environment, it is critical that nurses are poised to articulate a philosophy of nursing that sets forth values, beliefs about nursing, the relationship of nursing, and the environment of nursing (Parker, 2005). Philosophy is concerned with the purpose of human life, the nature of the being, and the theory and limits of knowledge. Generating new knowledge is a common goal of both science and philosophy (Fawcett, 1999, 2012; Silva, 1977).

Nursing, as an art and a science, reflects all the ways of knowing (ANA, 2015b p. 17). Knowing is a cognitive process, and there are four fundamental patterns of knowing: empirics, personal, esthetics, and ethical (Carper, 1978; 1992). These patterns don't exist in isolation, but rather are used in combination in varying degrees depending on the nursing situation. There are three facets to nursing knowledge: ontology (study of being, what is or what exists), epistemology (study of knowledge or ways of knowing), and methodology (acquiring new knowledge) (Powers & Knapp, 2011).

Nurses, as scientists, rely on qualitative and quantitative evidence to guide policies and practices, but also as a way of identifying the nurse's impact on the health outcomes of healthcare consumers (ANA, 2015b, p. 13). Research is a systematic inquiry that uses rigorous methodology to answer or solve a problem as well as to validate or refine existing knowledge and generate new knowledge. "Nurse researchers conduct research that is relevant to communities of interest and guided by participation of these communities in identifying research problems, and that strives to benefit patients, society, and professional practice" (ANA, 2010). Nursing research involves the design and implementation of a study that is important to nursing (e.g., practice, education, administration, and informatics) (Polit & Beck, 2008). The main reason to conduct nursing research is to advance nursing knowledge that can be applied to practice (Smith & Parker, 2013). The practice of nursing is rooted in evidence-based knowledge (ANA, 2015b, p. 18).

Evidence-based practice is a lifelong problem-solving process that incorporates best available evidence, with clinical expertise, and considers patient/family values, wishes, and preferences for clinical decision making. Nephrology nurses should address the gap between research and practice by implementing evidence-based practice that measures clinical outcomes, thus supporting nephrology nurses' essential role in healthcare redesign (Hain & Kear, 2015).

Much of nursing practice is based on a critical thinking framework known as the nursing process that comprises assessment, diagnosis, outcomes identification, planning, implementation, and evaluation. Evidence-based competencies support the nursing process. There are similarities between the nursing process and the evidence-based practice process. Both can generate clinical outcomes that support quality and effective care that consider safety and person-centered care.

The art of nursing is based on a framework of caring and respect for human dignity. A compassionate approach to patient care carries an obligation to provide that care competently. Competent care is provided and accomplished through independent practice and collaborative partnerships. Collaboration may be with other colleagues or the individuals seeking support or assistance with their healthcare needs. Central to the nursing practice is the art of caring, which is represented by the interpersonal relationship that the nurse establishes with the patient.

Nursing Theories

"All professional disciplines have a body of knowledge consisting of theories, research, and methods of inquiry and practice. Theories are patterns that guide the thinking about, being, and doing of nursing" (Smith & Parker, 2013, p. 7). Nephrology nursing practice should be grounded in nursing theory. Nursing theory provides structure and organization to nursing knowledge, as well as a systematic means of collecting data to describe, explain, and predict nursing practice. Nursing theory should be used in the development of policies and procedures, training and education, clinical information systems, quality improvement programs, and professional development programs. Nursing theories are classified as *grand theories*, *middle-range theories*, and *practice theories*.

Grand theories are complex and broad in scope and they attempt to explain broad areas within a discipline such as adaptive systems, self-care deficits, unitary human beings, human becoming, or health as expanding consciousness (Smith & Parker, 2013). Middle-range theories are often more appropriate for empirical testing (can be operationalized). They may be rooted in grand theories or conceptual models. Practice level theories have limited scope and are used within a specific range of nursing situations (Smith & Parker, 2013).

It is sometimes difficult to decide when, where, and how to apply nursing theories. Nursing theories based on human needs, nursing process, caring, competency, and self-care may be adapted easily to nephrology nursing. Five of the nursing theorists and brief synopses of their theories are particularly applicable to nephrology nursing and are discussed below.

Dr. Patricia Benner (1984) created a model of nurses developing knowledge, skills, and understanding of how to care for patients through education and experience. This model provides a framework for assessing nurses' needs at different stages of professional growth. Benner's model can be applied to an orientation and mentoring program that addresses the level of nursing experience in caring for individuals with kidney disease.

The five stages are as follows:

1. *Novice*: The beginner nurse with no experience. At this stage the nurse has limited ability to practice without support from more experienced nurses. The nurse practices from general context-free rules that are independent of specific cases.
2. *Advanced Beginner*: The nurse is relatively new but has demonstrated knowledge and skill and has gained some experience that enables

him/her to identify recurring meanings to the nursing situation. The clinical experiences help guide actions. The nurse can practice with occasional supportive cues.

3. *Competent*: The nurse has experience in a similar position for 2 to 3 years and is able to demonstrate efficiency and has mastery over critical thinking skills. The nurse takes a more holistic approach to clinical decision making.
4. *Proficient*: The nurse is able to perceive the situation as a whole and able to apply meaning to the situation in the establishment of long-term goals. The nurse recognizes the need to revise plans based on the changing situations. The experience gained helps the nurse learn from past experiences and know what to expect in certain situations.
5. *Expert*: The nurse is no longer solely relying on rules and guidelines to connect the parts and determine appropriate actions but rather possesses an intuitive grasp on the situation and is able to focus on the relevant issues. The nurse's performance is fluid, flexible, and able to adapt to the situation as it evolves.

Jean Watson's model of human care focuses on the interpersonal relationship between the nurse and patient. Watson highlights the role of the nurse in defining the patient as a unique human being and emphasizes the importance of the connections between the nurse and patient. Nephrology nursing is moving from disease-focused care to person-centered care where the individual is cared for within a healing-caring environment. Watson's transpersonal caring–healing framework can guide interventions and nursing research. The following essential concepts are:

- The whole caring–healing consciousness is contained within a single caring moment.
- The one caring and the one being cared for are interconnected.
- Human caring and healing processes (or the noncaring, nonhealing consciousness of the nurse) are communicated to the one being cared for.

Madeline Leininger's theory of cultural care diversity and universality addresses care for people from a broad range of cultures, and comprises five theoretical assumptions on caring:

- Care is essential for human growth and survival, and to face death.
- There can be no curing without caring.
- Expressions of care vary among all cultures of the world.
- Therapeutic nursing care can only occur when cultural care values, expressions, or practices are known and used explicitly.
- Nursing is a transcultural care profession and discipline.

A growing ethnically and culturally diverse population living with kidney disease demands that nephrology nurses embrace the uniqueness of each person. Strategies aimed at improving health outcomes of people with kidney disease can be guided by Leininger's theory.

Dorothea Orem's self-care deficit nursing theory (SCDNT) is based on the belief that humans require continuous and deliberate inputs into themselves and interaction with their environment to remain alive and to function. Individuals living with kidney disease are often expected to engage in self-management activities that promote health. Self-care is central to Orem's theory, and associated constructs can support interventions that promote self-management.

The theory purports five methods of helping:

- Acting for and doing for others
- Guiding others
- Supporting another
- Providing an environment promoting personal development in relation to meeting future demands
- Teaching another

The dialysis arena is one area of nursing practice in which the application of this theory would be appropriate because it is crucial for patients to be actively involved in self-care (Simmons, 2009).

Pender's Health Promotion Model "is a guide for exploration of the complex biopsychological processes that motivate individuals to engage in health behaviors directed toward the enhancement of health" (Pender, 1996, p. 51). One of the main assumptions is that people have the ability to determine their own destiny, and perceived self-efficacy is key to the development of desired outcomes or actions. In one study in which Pender's model guided a kidney disease education program, participants who gained CKD self-management knowledge and increased self-efficacy were able to engage in self-management that helped slow the progression of the disease (Enworom & Tabi, 2015).

The aforementioned theories provide exemplars for nephrology nursing research and practice. These are not meant to be inclusive of all the potential theories that may apply to nephrology nursing, but rather demonstrate the essential role theories have in providing a meaningful direction for nephrology nursing research and practice.

Evolution of Nephrology Nursing

As early as 1915, nursing literature mentions the care of patients with kidney disease. In the early stages of nephrology nursing, most nursing authors focused on the physical care of these patients, including:

- Recording intake and output
- Controlling the diet
- Maintaining elimination of wastes through the gastrointestinal tract
- Providing sufficient rest
- Preventing infection
- Decreasing muscle activity to minimize the production of metabolic wastes
- Keeping the patient comfortable

The Artificial Kidney (Coleman & Merrill, 1952) was the first article published in the nursing literature to describe the role of the nurse in dialysis. In 1960, the arteriovenous shunt was developed, enabling the long-term treatment of kidney failure with hemodialysis. As the number of patients on hemodialysis increased and the techniques advanced, it was no longer feasible or necessary for physicians to remain at the bedside during the treatments. Nurses assumed responsibility for the majority of hemodialysis procedures (Hoffart, 1989).

Peritoneal dialysis, as a therapy for chronic kidney disease, began in the 1970s with technique improvements developed by Doctors Boen, Oreopoulis, Moncrief, Lasker, and Tenckhoff. Nephrology nurses had to initiate, maintain, and monitor the patient and the therapy. This involved recording the intake and output, handling drainage problems, and keeping the patient safe. In 1978, the FDA approved the continuous ambulatory peritoneal dialysis (CAPD) technique system developed by Baxter.

Nephrology nurses began teaching individuals with CKD how to perform peritoneal dialysis in their homes as a branch of home dialysis training. In 1981, a prototype of an automatic peritoneal dialysis machine, known as the cycler, was designed. It allowed patients to transition from manual exchanges of dialysate solution during the day to an automated process where the machine fills and drains solution from the patient. This technique is known as continuous cycling peritoneal dialysis (CCPD) (Guest, 2014).

Throughout history, the possibility of transplanting organs and tissues from one body to another has been intriguing. More than 50 years have passed since the first long-term successful kidney transplant was performed. Nephrology nurses have been involved in every phase of the procedure. From organ procurement and pretransplant workup to the postoperative phase, nephrology nurses are active members of the interdisciplinary team. The early work of nephrology nurses caring for patients with kidney transplants greatly contributed to the development of other transplant nursing programs.

Congress enacted the Social Security Amendments of 1972 (P.L.92-603) of Section 299I. This legislation authorized Medicare entitlement for individuals with a diagnosis of chronic renal failure who were fully or currently insured under Social Security. It also authorized coverage for the spouse and dependent children of fully or currently insured individuals. Persons with a diagnosis of chronic renal failure were "deemed to be disabled" for purposes of coverage under Parts A and B of Medicare (Rettig, 1991).

Nephrology nursing, as a specialty, continued to expand as kidney replacement therapy (hemodialysis and peritoneal dialysis) and transplant units were established throughout the United States. The equipment-dependent methods of treatment (hemodialysis and peritoneal dialysis) threatened to dehumanize patients and take away their control. The patients and their families felt the stress of being dependent on a dialysis machine, financial concerns, strict medical regimens, and the stress resulting from changes in lifestyle (Hoffart, 1989). Nephrology nurses work to personalize the experience and to provide holistic care.

Nephrology Nursing Process

Nephrology nurses use the nursing process in providing care to patients with kidney disease. The nursing process comprises assessment, diagnosis, outcomes identification, planning, implementation, and evaluation. Each phase of the nursing process interacts with and is influenced by the other phases.

Assessment

The nephrology registered nurse/advanced practice registered nurse (APRN) collects comprehensive data pertinent to the healthcare consumer's health and/or the situation.

Diagnosis

The nephrology registered nurse/advanced practice registered nurse analyzes the assessment data to determine the diagnoses or the issues.

Outcomes Identification

The nephrology registered nurse/advanced practice registered nurse identifies expected outcomes for a plan individualized to the healthcare consumer or the situation.

Planning

The nephrology registered nurse/advanced practice registered nurse develops an individualized plan that prescribes strategies and alternatives to attain expected outcomes.

Implementation

The nephrology registered nurse implements the identified plan, coordinates care delivery, and employs strategies to promote health and a safe environment. The advanced practice registered nurse specializing in nephrology provides consultation to influence the identified plan, enhance the abilities of others, and effect change. The advanced practice registered nurse performs and reviews procedures and assists in development of protocols, coordinates referrals, uses prescriptive authority, and provides treatments and therapies in accordance with state and federal laws and regulations. The nephrology advanced practice registered nurse participates with the interdisciplinary team in the development of the comprehensive care plan.

Evaluation

The nephrology registered nurse/advanced practice registered nurse evaluates progress toward attainment of outcomes and manages changes to help patients meet their goals.

Differentiated Roles and Settings of Nephrology Nursing Practice

The majority of nephrology nursing practice focuses on the patient population with identified kidney disease. Nephrology nurses work in a variety of multidisciplinary and interdisciplinary environments. Nephrology nurses also practice within the community in the prevention and identification of kidney disease. Patient care is provided through a team approach involving nurses, patient care technicians, dialysis technologists, biomedical technicians, social workers, dietitians, physicians, and medical directors. The nephrology registered nurse provides clinical supervision of the licensed practical/vocational nurse (LPN/LVN) and patient care technicians (PCT) in accordance with state practice acts and the Centers for Medicare and Medicaid Services (CMS) Conditions for Coverage (CfCs) regulations (CMS, 2008). Wherever they practice, nephrology nurses use critical thinking to respond to the needs of patients with kidney disease. They are mindful of resource utilization through the implementation of strategies and interventions that provide optimal outcomes most appropriate to the healthcare consumer or situation.

The practice of nephrology nursing may include, but is not limited to, those practices listed below.

Staff Nurse, Hospital, or Outpatient Settings

The nephrology nurse may work in the inpatient or outpatient setting. Inpatient includes hospital units caring for patients with acute kidney injury (AKI), kidney disease, and transplant. The outpatient setting may include freestanding facilities, physician offices, and CKD clinics. These nephrology nurses focus in the areas of hemodialysis, peritoneal dialysis, transplant, organ recovery, quality management, infectious diseases, case management, CKD, and diabetic teaching.

Chronic Kidney Disease Management

One of the nephrology nurse's primary roles is to educate patients with kidney disease about their disease, treatment options, and health promotion. Nephrology nurses also guide patients and their families on strategies and interventions to prevent the progression of their kidney disease. The nephrology APRN can be reimbursed from Medicare for specific CKD Kidney Education for individuals with CKD stage 4 (CMS, 2009).

Advanced Practice in Nephrology Nursing

The nephrology advanced practice registered nurse (APRN) provides care for patients along the continuum of kidney disease and in all treatment modalities. APRNs are employed in the inpatient and/or outpatient setting with the APRN functioning as clinician, consultant, educator, and researcher.

APRNs in nephrology require substantial analytical knowledge and skills in nephrology nursing and the application and advancement of knowledge and skills in providing expert care to individuals diagnosed with kidney disease, their families, and the community at large. This advanced practice may include the roles of primary care provider, coordinator, consultant, educator, researcher, and administrator.

Consistent with ANA's *Nursing's Social Policy Statement and the Consensus Model for APRN Regulation: Licensure, Accreditation, Certification & Education* (APRN Consensus Work Group, 2008), the minimum requirements for an APRN with specialization in nephrology are graduate level preparation and certification in an APRN role and at least one population focus, including family/individual across the life span, adult/gerontology, neonatal, pediatrics, women's health/gender related, and/or psychiatric/mental health. The APRN with a specialty in nephrology may have additional didactic and clinical course work and experiences in that area.

The APRN prescribes in accordance to state and federal regulations. The APRN uses specific pharmacologic knowledge and experience to adjust medications as indicated for the patient with kidney disease. The APRN participates in the development and assessment of medication protocols.

Nephrology nurses practicing at the advanced level must be able to assess, diagnose, theorize, and analyze complex clinical and nonclinical problems related to the actual or potential diagnosis of kidney disease. In addition, advanced practice denotes the ability to consider a wide range of theory and research relevant to understanding kidney disease-related problems and the ability to select and justify the application of the most meaningful theory or research to assist in problem solving. The APRN contributes knowledge of nephrology nursing research to interdisciplinary workgroups to assure evidence-based guidelines are incorporated into nephrology nursing practice.

The APRN may serve as the healthcare provider to an individual diagnosed with kidney disease, their family, and the community. As a care coordinator, the advanced practice role involves the expert use of the application of change process with the interdisciplinary nephrology care team to determine and achieve realistic healthcare goals for the particular individual, the family, and/or an entire community, while guiding the patient through the healthcare system. The consultant role in advanced nephrology nursing practice involves providing expert advice about nephrology to colleagues, allied health personnel, and healthcare consumers. The educator role is exemplified by the assessment of learning needs, design, curriculum development and assessment, implementation, and evaluation of educational activities. The role of the researcher requires skills in the use of the research process, which include the ability to identify current researchable problems in nephrology nursing, collaborate in research, and evaluate and implement research findings that affect patient care or nephrology nursing. The administrative role involves use of the managerial process to promote a practice environment that reduces environmental health risks for the nephrology nurse, the patient, and the public.

The Clinical Nurse Leader

The Clinical Nurse Leader (CNL) is a nursing role developed by the American Association of Colleges and Nursing (AACN). AACN launched the CNL initiative in response to the call from the Institute of Medicine (IOM) and others to enhance the way nurses are educated and employed in the practice setting. The CNL is prepared for direct clinical leadership at the point of care to insure that care delivery is safe, evidence-based, and targeted toward optimal quality outcomes (Reid & Dennison, 2011).

The CNL in nephrology is a master's prepared nurse leader at the point of care who focuses on care coordination and transitions of care of individuals with kidney disease or acute kidney injury (AKI). The CNL engages in quality improvement, implementation of best practice based on best available evidence, and outcome measures within a microsystem (e.g., dialysis center, critical care unit). As a team leader, the CNL engages in interdisciplinary communication with other professionals, patients, families, caregivers, and unlicensed personnel to achieve quality patient outcomes.

Case Management

The nephrology nurse case manager oversees the quality, outcome, availability, and cost of patient care. Patient advocacy and continuity of care are two vital components of this role. Case managers coordinate care for patients in various settings such as before and after organ transplant, transitioning patients from CKD stage 3 to start of dialysis, and patients on dialysis who are managed in different settings from acute to long-term care. In this role, the case manager may also have development and administrative responsibilities for a particular program, such as a transplant manager. The establishment of ESCOs (ESRD Seamless Care Organizations) under the Medicare benefit has included the case manager role to help meet outcomes set in these comprehensive care models.

Education

Many opportunities are available for nurses in nephrology education. The majority of nephrology education is provided by nephrology nurse educators in dialysis facilities. This role is an integral part of staff training and development. The nephrology nurse educator provides patient education using diversified training strategies. Some of the tools available to the nurse educator are interactive training programs, gaming, and Internet sites. The nephrology nurse educator is a valuable resource for facility and hospital staff, nurses from other disciplines, patient educators, and community outreach. In the academic setting, nephrology nurse educators may choose to teach undergraduate nursing, master's, or doctoral level programs.

Management

Nephrology nurses with leadership skills are ideal for the many management and administrative positions in both the inpatient and outpatient settings. Managers lead teams in all modalities. This may include managing an outpatient chronic hemodialysis center or a home training center. Nephrology nurse managers working in the acute setting lead the acute dialysis team while collaborating with hospital departments. Managers in the transplant environment may oversee the transplant center as well as the renal/kidney transplant unit. Responsibilities of this role may include budgetary planning and monitoring, inventory control, regulatory compliance, contract negotiation, oversight of staff education and competency programs, patient education and training, patient engagement and experience, and continuous quality improvement programs.

Research and Evidence-Based Practice

As nephrology nursing embraces evidence-based practice, the importance of nursing research to inform practice becomes more apparent. Nephrology nurses should engage in evidence-based practice as they translate the best available evidence into practice, while incorporating nursing expertise and patient/family values and wishes into clinical decision making. Nursing research and evidence-based practice specific to nephrology are crucial in the ongoing development and advancement of the specialty.

Corporate/Government

Corporate employers include manufacturers and distributors of dialysis equipment and related products, as well as pharmaceutical companies. Nephrology nurses may be directly involved in the development of equipment and products. In government settings, nurses are involved on the local, state, and federal levels and lead ESRD facility surveys. Nephrology nurses are also involved in responding to government policy changes such as Conditions for Coverage or National Quality Forum (NQF) measures.

Nursing Informatics

Nursing informatics requires nephrology nursing contributions. In this role, the nephrology nurse is responsible for managing and communicating data as well as the development and implementation of electronic medical record systems using information technology guidelines. Informatics is used in providing data to federal and state regulators and agencies such as CMS, Crown Web, ESRD Networks, and state health departments. Patient and facility level data are collected and shared with various agencies for quality reporting. Data collected is also used by CMS for payment schedules based on meeting specific quality indicators.

Miscellaneous areas for nephrology nursing contribution include legislation and regulatory affairs, professional associations, home health, and palliative and hospice nursing.

There are increasing requirements from regulatory agencies to report "in-time" data on the nephrology workforce. This can present a problem to the specialty as workforce data are not a required reporting point for dialysis centers. The data collection relies on voluntary reporting from private and hospital-owned dialysis organizations sharing their workforce data. Developing such a tool would add additional costs to both human and financial resources.

It remains difficult to determine the exact number of nephrology registered nurses in practice today. A snapshot of the membership profile of the specialty's professional association, the American Nephrology Nurses Association (ANNA), may provide insight into the areas of practice and positions held by association members. Total membership as of 2016 was 8,751. The ANNA membership profile is updated annually and available to the members on the ANNA website (www.annanurse.org).

Areas of Practice (multiple – % total list)

	Count	Percent
Acute Care	2,928	33.46%
Chronic Hemodialysis	4,703	53.74%
Chronic Kidney Disease	2,041	23.32%
Conservative Management	263	3.01%
CRRT	844	9.64%
Home Therapies	794	9.07%
Medical Surgical Unit	466	5.33%
Nursing Education	864	9.87%
Pediatric Nephrology	406	4.64%
Peritoneal Dialysis	1,914	21.87%
Research	231	2.64%
Therapeutic Apheresis	491	5.61%
Transplantation	536	6.13%
Other	518	5.92%

Primary Position

	Count	Percent
Administration	591	7.24%
Case Manager	120	1.47%
Clinical Nurse Specialist	196	2.40%
Coordinator	358	4.39%
Education	687	8.42%
Head Nurse/Supervisor	1,169	14.32%
Nurse Practitioner	426	5.22%
Retired	114	1.40%
Staff/Clinical Nurse	3,934	48.20%
Other	566	6.94%

For the most recent statistical information, go to https://www.annanurse.org/about/association/fact-sheet

Education and Professional Development

Continuing Education

Registered nurses receive general education on kidney disease in their basic nursing education programs. Additional education for registered nurses interested in nephrology should include content related to acute kidney injury (AKI), patient management, fluid and electrolytes, acid-base balance, pharmacology considerations, and complications.

The standardization of training is an issue as it is within any specialty. The majority of training and education is delivered at the facility level. The APRN with a specialty in nephrology most often has been educationally prepared and certified as a clinical nurse specialist or nurse practitioner within a specific recognized track that does not include nephrology. Formal educational programs to prepare APRNs with a specialty in nephrology nursing are limited. The majority of nephrology APRNs have been mentored by a nephrologist or APRN in the field.

Nephrology registered nurses are accountable for judgments made and actions taken in the course of their nursing practice. Therefore, the process of continuing education is imperative. Since the 1950s, the fast-paced evolution of nephrology care has made continuing education (CE) critical to the success of nephrology nurses and the patients they care for. This process was formally recognized when ANNA was first created and later when nephrology nursing certification was developed. Recertification requirements include attendance or participation in nephrology-specific continuing education programs or online activities.

ANNA recognizes the importance of continuing education and offers scholarships that provide funding to support members in their pursuit of higher education. In addition, ANNA offers numerous online educational programs on their Prolibraries site (http://www.prolibraries.com/anna), live seminars, teleconferences, and their volunteer leadership education workshop (VLW).

The National Kidney Foundation (NKF) hosts the Council of Nephrology Nurses and Technicians (CNNT) and the Council of Advanced Practitioners (CAPS) that function as a professional membership council within NKF.

Professional Organization

The American Nephrology Nurses Association (ANNA) is the specialty's professional association. ANNA was founded and has supported nephrology nurses since 1968. Nephrology nurses have consistently supported the endeavors of the organization as it continues to meet their professional needs. The association's mission and values have been updated and revised to reflect the changes in nephrology nursing practice. The current mission and core beliefs are noted below (for the full strategic plan, go to https://www.annanurse.org/download/reference/association/strategicPlan.pdf).

Mission. ANNA promotes excellence in and appreciation of nephrology nursing so we can make a positive difference for people with kidney disease (ANNA, 2016; https://annanurse.org/about).

The ANNA published Core Beliefs include:

1. Nephrology nurses have an opportunity and responsibility to enhance the quality of care delivered to people with kidney disease.
2. As an organization, we have the responsibility to provide sound educational programs necessary to develop, maintain, and augment competence in practice, and that we as individual practitioners have the responsibility to continue to deepen our knowledge, sharpen our skills, and develop our competencies.
3. ANNA must support research to develop evidence-based practice, as well as to advance nursing science, and that as individual members, we must support, participate in, and apply evidence-based research that advances our own skills, as well as nursing science.
4. We must support and engage in collaboration that results in higher quality patient care and more cost-effective healthcare delivery.
5. We benefit as an organization and as individuals when we embrace and nurture diversity in all of its dimensions.
6. Nurses must be respected in the workplace, and ways of demonstrating this respect are to support them in their professional growth and employ them at their highest level of education and training.
7. ANNA must provide nurses with leadership opportunities, and nurses need to seize opportunities to develop and polish their leadership skills.
8. We benefit intellectually and spiritually when we socialize together.

Publications. Additional resources published through the years have enabled ANNA to establish itself as the voice for the nephrology nursing specialty. In 1972, the association published its first *Standards of Clinical Practice*, which addressed hemodialysis, followed in 1974–75 with *Standards of Clinical Practice for Transplantation*, and in 1975–76 with *Standards of Clinical Practice for Peritoneal Dialysis*. Over the years, the standards have been revised to include updated information, structured standards, patient teaching, patient outcomes, and new therapeutic modalities. This eighth edition of ANNA's *Nephrology Nursing Scope and Standards of Practice* incorporates competencies for both the registered nurse, graduate-level nurse, and the advanced practice registered nurse working in nephrology.

The *Core Curriculum for Nephrology Nursing* was first published in 1987 and is now in its sixth edition. The textbook, *Contemporary Nephrology Nursing*, was first published in 1998, with its third edition in 2017. In addition to books, the association has published monographs on therapeutic modalities, rehabilitation, and disaster nursing, as well as publications on topics specific to the nephrology nursing roles, research, professional development, and quality assurance.

Position papers developed and published by ANNA have also played an important role in the specialty. Position statements represent succinct summaries of ANNA's stance on a variety of issues for the purpose of influence, advocacy, and/or clarification. Beginning in 1977 with a position paper on the role of the hemodialysis technician, the association has delineated its positions and those of nephrology nursing on a variety of issues including, but not limited to, the scope of practice of nephrology nursing, delegation, certification, and health policy issues. For the most current position statements, go to https://www.annanurse.org/advocacy/resources-and-tools/position-statements.

ANNA endorses the recommendations of other organizations that support concerns that affect nephrology nursing or our patients. To find more information on these endorsements, go to https://www.annanurse.org/advocacy/endorsements and https://www.annanurse.org/advocacy/health-policy/legislative-priorities.

Certification

In 1986, the ANNA Board of Directors voted to pursue the development of a process to certify proficiency in nephrology nursing practice. With the assistance of the National League for Nursing Testing Service, an ANNA certification ad hoc committee developed a criterion-referenced examination. The exam was designed to ascertain if a nurse who took the exam met the established standard of proficiency in nephrology nursing.

The first test was administered in 1987. In that year, the Certification Ad Hoc Committee evolved to become the Nephrology Nursing Certification Board (NNCB). NNCB was established as a separate corporation with its own bylaws, officers, and board of directors. In 2000, NNCB changed its name to the Nephrology Nursing Certification Commission (NNCC) to reflect a broader scope of certification and recertification activities. The NNCC model of the certification examination for the specialty of nephrology nursing is based on the Dreyfus model of skill acquisition, as adapted by Patricia Benner.

The 2016 ANNA membership profile (www.annanurse.org) reflects the certification status of its membership as the following:

Certification Status (multiple)

	Count	Percent
CNN	2,542	29.05%
CDN	610	6.97%
CCHT	233	2.66%
CNN-NP	50	0.57%
CNNe	36	0.41%
CCRN	126	1.44%
CDE	12	0.14%
Certified by ANA	81	0.93%
Other	690	7.88%
	4,380	

Key

CNN certified nephrology nurse
CDN certified hemodialysis nurse
CCHT certified clinical hemodialysis technician
CNN-NP certified nephrology nurse practitioner
CNNe certified nephrology nurse emeritus
CCRN certified critical care registered nurse
CDE certified diabetes educator

Health Policy Involvement

Advocacy is one of the strategic issues identified in ANNA's Strategic Plan. Over the years, ANNA and its members have actively participated in the legislative and regulatory arenas. ANNA established its Government Relations Committee in 1981, published its first Legislative Policy Statement in November 1983 (Parker, 1998), developed a state legislative representative program in 1988, and established a legislative office in Washington, DC, in 1989. Today, ANNA maintains a Health Policy Agenda and a Health Policy Statement, which are reviewed annually.

ANNA's Health Policy Specialty Practice Network (SPN) employs a national strategy to identify, monitor, and address issues that could affect nursing practice, especially nephrology nursing practice, and/or patients. This strategy crosses the local, state, and national levels.

In 2003, ANNA held its first End-Stage Renal Disease (ESRD) Education Day. This was a nationwide effort to inform lawmakers about the urgent need to modernize Medicare and help save patients' lives. Lawmakers at the federal, state, and local levels were invited to visit their local dialysis units and learn more about the challenges their constituents face. This education day has evolved into the Kidney Disease Awareness and Education Week (KDAE Week) with increased visits from lawmakers throughout the year. ANNA hosts a biannual Health Policy Workshop where members learn about health policy issues and have an opportunity to visit Capitol Hill. In conjunction with the workshop, ANNA hosts a Virtual Lobby Day that allows members unable to attend the Health Policy Workshop to contact their legislative members via email and phone to lend a voice to those representing ANNA on the Hill.

ANNA maintains the ANNA legislative center where nephrology nurses can quickly identify their legislative representative and communicate electronically on critical issues. ANNA was actively involved in responding to changes in the Medicare and Medicaid programs: the Conditions for Coverage for End-Stage Renal Disease Facilities (CfC) and implementation of the Medicare prospective payment system (PPS) for services to patients with end-stage renal disease (ESRD). ANNA has participated each year in the comments process for the ESRD Prospective Payment System (PPS) and the ESRD Quality Incentive Program (QIP).

The current health policy agenda priorities include monitoring of policies related to the PPS, QIP, and patient education programs; collaborating with entities that define nursing-related quality measures; endorsing health policy initiatives that promote organ donation, increase transplantation, prevent chronic kidney disease, and monitor effects of new laws and regulations that impact the ESRD program and its beneficiaries. ANNA also monitors nursing and general healthcare issues and has responded by supporting increased funding for the Nursing Workforce Development programs and appropriations for the National Institute for Nursing Research (NINR). In addition, ANNA encourages and maintains promotion of safe workplace initiatives, federal and state nursing practice issues and their effects on nephrology nursing, and healthcare reform proposals.

ANNA continues to support the need to ensure healthcare consumer safety and access to APRNs by aligning education, accreditation, licensure, and certification as shown in the Consensus Model for APRN Regulation: Licensure, Accreditation, Certification, and Education (APRN JDG, 2008). ANNA endorses the specialty certification of the certified nephrology nurse practitioner (CNN-NP).

Healthy Work Environments

The importance of examining the role of the nephrology nurse is critical in bringing about positive patient outcomes and improving the quality and safety of patient care. Nephrology nursing practice issues are related to a safe workplace, nursing excellence, and safe practice. It is important to gain a clear understanding of the work environment factors that encourage and discourage the recruitment and retention of qualified nephrology nurses, especially in freestanding dialysis units. Evidence from magnet hospital research reveals aspects of the dialysis work environment that may contribute to the shortage of nurses in the hemodialysis unit (Thomas-Hawkins,

Flynn, & Clarke, 2008). Additional discussion regarding this study and its impact on patient care can be found in the article by Yoder, Xin, Norris, and Yan (2013).

With this in mind, ANNA funded a study to determine the impact of nephrology registered nurses on patient outcomes. Findings from the study support the nursing organization's and outcomes model proposition that nephrology RN staffing levels have a significant impact on patient outcomes. The mean patient-to-RN ratio was 9.58 patients per RN: 25% of nurses cared for 4.61 patients or less and 31% of nurses cared for 12 patients or more. Patient-to-RN ratios of 12 or more patients per RN were significantly associated with higher odds of frequent occurrences of shortened and skipped dialysis treatments and patient complaints compared to RNs with the lowest patient-to-RN ratios (i.e., 4.61 or fewer patients per RN) (Thomas-Hawkins et al., 2008). Two limitations of the study were the wide variation in RN staffing levels and the use of nurse-reported data.

Whether they come from individual corporations or from regulatory agencies, nephrology nurses are constantly faced with the possible implementation of arbitrary staffing ratios and other workforce and workplace constraints. Nephrology nurses need to continue to be diligent in their awareness of pending regulations impacting practice.

In 2014, the first national study of Patient Safety Culture in Nephrology Nursing Practice was conducted on behalf of ANNA (Ulrich & Kear, 2014a). The results indicated that the safety of both the nephrology nurse and the patient with kidney disease was being compromised. The investigators concluded that nephrology nurses are responsible for providing safe patient care as well as creating an environment in which others can provide safe patient care (Ulrich & Kear, 2014b).

Nursing excellence and establishing best practice in all areas of nephrology nursing practice are a focus for the specialty. Interdisciplinary evidence-based guidelines for CKD care are available as a reference to all nephrology practitioners from the following associations:

- National Kidney Foundation Kidney Disease Outcomes Quality Initiative (NKF KDOQI) (https:/www.kidney.org/professionals/guidelines)
- Renal Physicians Association (RPA) (http:/www.renalmd.org/page.aspx?id=2544)
- Kidney Disease: Improving Global Outcomes (KDIGO) (http://kdigo.org/home/guidelines)
- American Nephrology Nurses Association (ANNA) (https://annanurse.org)

Nephrology nursing continues to be actively involved as future guidelines are developed. Nephrology nurses must advocate for policies and procedures that address the issue of workplace safety.

Ethics

Nephrology registered nurses are bound by a professional code of ethics as described by the American Nursing Association (ANA, 2015a) and regulate themselves as individuals through peer review of practice. With this guidance from ANA, nephrology nurses are encouraged to use these interpretive statements for each of the nine provisions described in the **ANA Code of Ethics** (below).

PROVISION NUMBER *The nephrology nurse:*	EXAMPLE
1. Practices with compassion and respect for the inherent dignity, worth, and unique attributes of individuals receiving nephrology care whether an individual, family, group, community, or population.	Elizabeth confides in John, her primary care nurse, that she wishes to stop dialysis after 6 years. She feels her quality of life is poor, yet her family will not allow her to discuss her feelings. John sits with her and listens as she expresses her concerns. He asks her permission to arrange a family meeting, which includes the renal social worker and APRN to help facilitate communication and support Elizabeth.
2. Primary commitment is to the nephrology patient, whether an individual, family, group, community or population.	Marie works in a facility serving an Orthodox Jewish community and has alternate treatment schedules to meet their religious observations on the Sabbath and other religious holidays. New employee orientation includes specific education regarding specific values and beliefs of the Orthodox community.
3. Promotes, advocates for, and protects the rights, health, and safety of the nephrology patient.	While reading a recent listserv post, Mark notes an FDA recall related to equipment in use at his facility and reports it immediately to the dialysis facility administrator.
4. Has authority, accountability, and responsibility for nursing practice; makes decisions; takes action consistent with the obligation to promote health and to provide optimal kidney replacement care.	Anna, an APRN, leads the CKD clinic held bimonthly at a local nephrologist's office. Anna guides the transition to dialysis by referring her patients for access placement and providing modality education, including advanced medical directive discussions. She also monitors for and manages complications as kidney disease progresses such as anemia, hypertension, and bone metabolism disorder. Her interventions help to slow progression to ESRD, and encourage transplant before dialysis and home therapies.

Continues on next page

PROVISION NUMBER *The nephrology nurse:*	EXAMPLE
5. Owes the same duties to self as to others, including the responsibility to promote health and safety, preserve wholeness of character and integrity, maintain competence, and continue personal and professional growth within the nephrology specialty.	Nephrology nurses participating with ANNA and collaborating with the Human Resources Program supported Rwandan nephrology nurses pursuing their MSc-N nephrology track degree by providing educational materials and online educational support developed by nephrology nurses in the United States (Mukamana et al., 2016).
6. Through individual and collective effort, establishes, maintains, and improves the ethical environment of the work setting and conditions of employment that are conducive to safe, quality KRT care.	Jen is a nurse manager who relies on Association for the Advancement of Medical Instrumentation (AAMI) and Centers for Medicare and Medicaid Services (CMS) guidelines to set up policies, procedures, and safety checks within her dialysis facility.
7. In all roles and settings, advances nephrology nursing as a profession through scholarly inquiry, professional nephrology nursing standards development, and the generation of nursing and health policy as it relates to kidney replacement therapies.	Jane is an educator for the dialysis department and used the *Nephrology Nursing Scope and Standards of Practice* to develop a competency checklist. She also leads a journal club, highlighting articles from the peer-reviewed ANNA *Nephrology Nursing Journal.*
8. Collaborates with other health professionals and public to protect human rights, promote health diplomacy, and reduce health disparities within kidney replacement therapy care.	The local ANNA chapter volunteers to participate in a National Kidney Foundation (NKF) Kidney Early Evaluation Program (KEEP) event twice a year (https://www.kidney.org/news/keep).
9. Collectively through its professional organization, articulates nephrology nursing values, maintains the integrity of the nephrology nursing profession, and integrates principles of social justice into nephrology nursing and kidney replacement care health policy.	ANNA has nursing volunteers who participate on the health policy committee representing nephrology concerns in the local and federal arenas. There is a nephrology nurse volunteer who sits on the Kidney Care Partners (KCP) committee (http://kidneycarepartners.com/about-kcp).

Ethics concerns arise from the necessity of making difficult decisions in the face of conflicting interests. Ethics is now considered an important component of the undergraduate and graduate nursing curriculum. Hospitals are establishing ethics committees to review policies and procedures and provide consultation. All research must be approved by some form of an ethics review board. Nephrology nurses face many ethical concerns, such as treatment withdrawal, appropriateness of care, futility of treatment, allocation of resources, and management of disruptive or nonadherent patients in all areas of nephrology care (predialysis care, dialysis, or transplant). Some nephrology nurses may have personal ethical issues related to providing care based on their own personal beliefs and values. Nephrology nurses should seek training and education available from professional organizations or from educational offerings.

Nephrology nurses regularly evaluate safety, effectiveness, and resources in the planning and delivery of care. Nephrology nurses recognize that resources are limited and often unequally distributed. Consequently, they try to achieve more equitable distribution and availability of healthcare services throughout the local community, the country, and the world.

The Centers for Disease Control and Prevention (CDC), the Public Health Department, and ANA are developing crisis standards to be followed during a large-scale disaster. The patient with kidney disease is vulnerable to decreasing healthcare resources not only in a large-scale disaster, but in the current healthcare environment constrained by budget shortfalls.

Professional Trends and Issues

Evidence-Based Practice and Research

Nursing research and evidence-based practice contribute to the body of knowledge and enhance patient outcomes. As professionals, nurses continually evaluate and apply nursing research findings. New knowledge is translated to patient care to promote effective and efficient care and improved patient outcomes. In addition, nurses need to ensure practice changes are based on current evidence. The nursing profession continually examines nursing practice. An example of this is the study of the freestanding dialysis unit nurse staffing levels, which has demonstrated that safe staffing is imperative to quality patient care. Nephrology nurses need to continue to determine the work environment factors that encourage or discourage the requirement and retention of qualified nurses in freestanding dialysis units (Thomas-Hawkins, Denno, Currier, & Wick, 2003).

Evidence-based practice has emerged as an essential aspect of advanced practice nursing. Doctorally prepared registered nurses take a scholarly approach to the discipline and are committed to advancing the profession. The *DNP* (doctor of nursing practice) prepared nephrology nurse places a greater emphasis on practice by translating evidence into practice and evaluating outcomes. *PhD* (doctor of philosophy) prepared nephrology nurses discover the gap in the evidence and conduct research that contributes to the advancement of the science of nephrology nursing.

Research opportunities for nephrology nursing include the following, but not limited to:

- Coordination of the transition of the patient to kidney replacement therapies
- Education of primary care clinician in the timing for referral of the kidney patient to nephrologists and vascular surgeons
- Use of the APRN in nephrology settings

Genetic Diversity

Genomics is the study of genes and their function with the purpose of understanding their structure of the genome, including mapping genes and sequencing DNA. Genomics looks at molecular mechanisms and the interplay of genes and environment. In 2005, a consensus panel of nurse leaders established the *Essential Nursing Competencies and Curricula for Genetics and Genomics*. In 2006, ANNA endorsed the document and agreed to incorporate genetics into nursing education and practice. Anderson-Fabry disease (AFD), polycystic kidney disease (PKD), medullary cystic kidney disease (MCKD) and Alport syndrome are examples of kidney diseases with known genetic connections. Emerging evidence supports the important contribution genomics play in chronic kidney disease among African Americans. Nephrology nurses play an essential role in helping patients understand what this means in disease prevention and health promotion as more genomic evidence becomes available.

Cultural Competence

Cultural competence in health care refers to the capacity to provide effective medical care to persons of varied backgrounds through use of appropriate knowledge, skills, attitudes, and behaviors. According to Cross, Bazron, Dennis, and Isaacs (1989):

- *Culture* refers to integrated patterns of human behavior that include the language, thoughts, communications, actions, customs, beliefs, values, and institutions of racial, ethnic, religious, or social groups.
- *Competence* implies having the capacity to function effectively as an individual and an organization within the context of the cultural beliefs, behaviors, and needs presented by consumers and their communities.

Developing cultural competence allows a practitioner to understand, communicate with, and effectively interact with people across cultures. Developing a culturally competent approach to provision of health care requires a patient-centered approach that will affect care given to individuals of any community, including those defined by gender, sexual orientation, and disability. Cultural competence includes four components (Sue, Arredondo, & McDavis, 1992):

1. Awareness of one's own cultural worldview.
2. Attitude toward cultural differences.
3. Knowledge of different cultural practices and worldviews.
4. Cross-cultural skills.

ESRD is more common among adults over 70 years of age. African Americans are about three and a half times more likely to develop ESRD than whites. Hispanics are about one and a half times more likely to develop ESRD than non-Hispanics (USRDS, 2013). Nephrology nurses need to develop strategies to produce positive health outcomes among all patient populations.

Technologic Advances

Technology offers the promise of creating a better work environment for nurses when it is designed and implemented in a manner that supports the nurses' work. Ideally, technology eliminates redundancy and duplication of documentation, and reduces probability of errors. The devices used in nephrology nursing are becoming increasingly complex. The nephrology registered nurse needs to have an additional skill set to work not only with specific dialysis equipment, but with the new and diverse electronic health record (EHR) and clinical documentation systems. Development of computerized programs that monitor patient outcomes have become commonplace.

Nephrology registered nurses need to be part of the planning and implementation of technology in the workplace. As healthcare resources become limited, the costs of technology need to be weighed against the benefit to patient care. The nephrology registered nurse needs to be represented when these decisions are made.

Technology can be used in research to improve data collection and analysis as well as to provide information on current patient demographics, comorbidities, and measuring outcomes. Computerized staffing models can provide the nephrology nurse with more time to interact with the patient. The incorporation of any technology, however, is not without risk, and it demands due diligence by nephrology nurses to consider the impact on the scope of nursing practice and the ethical and safety implications for healthcare consumers.

Nephrology Nurse Sensitive Outcomes

Quality of care is a multidimensional construct with three categories of quality indicators related to structure, processes, and outcomes of health care (Donabedian, 2005). *Structure indicators* refer to characteristics of the healthcare setting that affect a system's ability to provide services or resources. Examples include optimal staffing ratios or a CKD education program. *Process indicators* refer to the care that is actually being delivered. *Outcome indicators* involve the health status of the patient.

The identification of nephrology nursing sensitive quality indicators (NNSQI) is critical in measuring and demonstrating the positive impact nephrology nursing has on patient care and in fulfilling ANNA's commitment to advancing the nephrology nursing specialty. The Task Force on Nurse Sensitive Outcomes (TFNSO) was established to develop a definition of nephrology nurse sensitive quality indicators, recommendations to facilitate research and evidence-based nephrology nursing practice related to nephrology nursing sensitive quality indicators, and a linkage to ANNA's mission and the *Nephrology Nursing Scope and Standards of Practice*.

Nephrology nursing sensitive quality indicators are measures that reflect the structure, processes, and outcomes of care influenced by registered nurses (RNs). Structure is indicated by the nursing practice environment, RN skill mix, RN-to-patient ratios, and the education/certification of RNs. Process indicators measure aspects of nursing care, such as assessment, diagnosis, planning, intervention, and evaluation, as well as the surveillance and supervision of staff. Outcome indicators include patient outcomes, clinician outcomes, or provider outcomes sensitive to the quality or quantity of nursing care (ANNA, 2014).

Future of Nephrology Nursing

Despite a rising incidence of kidney disease, rates of kidney failure and related deaths are declining in the United States. Researchers at the United States Renal Data System (USRDS, 2015a) project that about 14% of U.S. adults have chronic kidney disease, which can progress to kidney failure. Because of an aging and overweight population, the rate of end-stage kidney disease is on the rise, according to USRDS. In the United States, there are over 26 million individuals with CKD markers, and millions of others are at risk.

In 2013, per patient per year (PPPY) costs reached $21,909 for Medicare CKD patients aged 65 and older, an 8.7% increase compared to 2012 ($20,162), but a decrease since 2010 ($22,440). The overall difference reflects both changes in average spending by stage (spending increased in all CKD stages from 2012), and the shift toward the less severe and less costly stages. Costs for patients with CKD stages 4–5 ($27,405) were 38.0% greater than costs for patients with CKD stages 1–2 ($19,859). Costs for Black/African-American patients exceeded those for White patients by

12.7%, somewhat lower than the 19.6% gap observed in 2010 (USRDS, 2015b).

Nephrology registered nurses specializing in the care of patients with kidney disease require a specific body of knowledge as well as complex technical skills. The care that was described in the literature decades ago still serves as the foundation for current care. However, the level of complexity has escalated. The number of patients is increasing. The average age of the patient is rising. The number of comorbidities has dramatically increased.

The impending shortage of nephrology nurses is less of a concern than the loss of the *experienced* nephrology nurse. The average age of the practicing nephrology nurse continues to increase as does the number of nephrology nurses retiring from the profession. Consequently, the economic and quality of care impacts are considerable. Nephrology nurses have many challenges to face in the future.

A commitment to nephrology nursing requires nurses to remain involved in continuous learning and be accountable for strengthening individual practice through varied practice settings as well as membership in and support of professional associations. The future will show us that

- Nephrology nursing will strengthen the formalized training and education process for the specialty. Formalized education programs in academic nursing programs for advanced practice registered nurses will be available in all areas of the country.
- Nephrology nursing will support the funding of nursing schools to recruit and retain adequate faculty to prepare registered nurses for practice.
- Nephrology nursing will continue to actively encourage nursing research that seeks to examine the specific characteristics of the nephrology work environments, how technology can be used to redesign nephrology workplace environments to meet the needs of patients and the nurses providing their care, and the impact of professional nursing care on patient outcomes.

As we face economic challenges, encroachment upon nephrology nursing practice remains a concern. Nephrology nurses underestimate the knowledge they bring to the interdisciplinary team and at times abdicate the leadership role to other disciplines. The future of nephrology nursing depends on the specialty to continue to advocate for the right to lead the interdisciplinary team through continued presence at the "decision-making table."

Nephrology nurses will continue to work independently and as members of coalitions at the state and federal levels to identify and respond to health policy issues that affect the practice of nephrology nurses and the individuals for whom they provide care.

Summary of the Nephrology Nursing Scope of Practice

The *Nephrology Nursing Scope and Standards of Practice, 8th Edition*, provides nephrology nursing with a method of defining the scope of its practice and a conduit for the evaluation of that practice. Moreover, this document serves as a guide in the identification of nephrology nurses' responsibilities to their profession, their colleagues, and the healthcare consumer. This publication can be used as a resource in the development of quality improvement programs, position descriptions, professional development programs, policies and procedures; it can also serve as a basis for the establishment of the legal standard of care.

Section 2 Nephrology Nursing Standards of Practice

Standards

A professional nursing organization has a responsibility to its members and to the public it serves to develop standards of practice. As the professional organization for all nephrology nurses, the American Nephrology Nurses Association (ANNA) has assumed the stewardship responsibility for developing and maintaining the standards of practice that apply to the specialty practice of nephrology nursing.

The standards of nephrology nursing practice are authoritative statements of the duties that all nephrology registered nurses are expected to perform competently. The standards contained in this document may serve to gauge the quality of care provided to patients with the understanding that the application of the standards is context dependent. The standards are subject to change with the dynamics of the nursing profession, nephrology practice, and local, state, and federal regulations. In addition, specific conditions and clinical circumstances may affect the application of the standards at a given time (e.g., during a natural disaster). The standards are subject to formal periodic review and revision.

The competencies that accompany each standard may be evidence of compliance with the corresponding standard. The list of competencies is not exhaustive. Whether a particular standard or competency applies depends upon the circumstances. For example, a nephrology nurse providing treatment to a comatose patient with acute kidney injury who has no family present still has a duty to collect comprehensive data pertinent to the patient's health (*Standard 1. Assessment*). However, that nurse would not be expected to assess family composition, history, and dynamics and the impact of those dynamics on the patient's health and wellness (*Standard 1. Assessment: Competencies*). The standard may include additional competencies for the graduate-level prepared nurse and/or the advanced practice registered nurse (APRN) specializing in nephrology nursing.

Definitions and Concepts Related to Competence (ANA, 2014)

- An individual who demonstrates competence is performing at an expected level.
- A competency is an expected level of performance that integrates knowledge, skills, abilities, and judgment.

- The integration of knowledge, skills, abilities, and judgment occurs in formal, informal, and reflective learning experiences.
- Knowledge encompasses thinking, understanding of science and humanities, professional standards of practice, and insights gained from context, practical experiences, personal capabilities, and leadership performance.
- Skills include psychomotor, communication, interpersonal, and diagnostic skills.
- Ability is the capacity to act effectively. It requires listening, integrity, knowledge of one's strengths and weaknesses, positive self-regard, emotional intelligence, and openness to feedback.
- Judgment includes critical thinking, problem solving, ethical reasoning, and decision making. (ANA, 2014)

Competence and Competency in Nephrology Nursing Practice

The competent practice of nephrology nursing can be influenced by the nature of the situation, which includes consideration of the setting, resources, and the person. Situations can either enhance or detract from the nephrology registered nurse's ability to perform. The nephrology registered nurse positively influences factors that facilitate and enhance competent practice. Similarly, the nephrology registered nurse seeks to overcome barriers that constrain competent practice. The expected level of performance reflects variability, depending upon context and the selected competence framework or model.

The ability to perform at the expected level requires a process of lifelong learning. Nephrology registered nurses must continually reassess their competencies and identify needs for additional knowledge, skills, personal growth, and integrative learning experiences.

Standards of Nephrology Nursing Practice

The standards of nephrology nursing practice describe a competent level of nursing care as demonstrated by the application of the nursing process. The standards may be used as the standard of care for the nephrology practitioner with the understanding that they are context dependent.

Standard 1 Assessment

The nephrology registered nurse collects pertinent data and information relative to the healthcare consumer's health or the situation.

Competencies

The nephrology registered nurse:

- Adheres to applicable federal, state, and local regulations for assessment criteria and frequency for healthcare consumers undergoing kidney replacement therapies (KRTs).
- Collects pertinent data including, but not limited to, demographics, social determinants of health, health disparities, and physical, functional, psychosocial, emotional, cognitive, sexual, cultural, age-related, environmental, spiritual/transpersonal, and economic assessments in a systematic, ongoing process with compassion and respect for the inherent dignity, worth, and unique attributes of the patient with kidney disease.
- Recognizes the importance of the assessment parameters identified by the World Health Organization (WHO), Healthy People 2020, or other organizations that influence nephrology nursing practice.
- Integrates knowledge from global and environmental factors into the assessment process.
- Elicits the healthcare consumer values, preferences, expressed and unexpressed needs, and knowledge of the healthcare situation.
- Engages the healthcare consumer and other interdisciplinary team members in holistic, culturally sensitive data collection.

- Identifies barriers to effective communication based on psychosocial, literacy, financial, and cultural considerations.
- Recognizes impact of one's own personal attitudes, values, and beliefs on the assessment process.
- Assesses the impact of family dynamics on health and wellness.
- Prioritizes data collection based on the healthcare consumer's immediate condition or the anticipated needs of the healthcare consumer or situation.
- Uses evidence-based assessment techniques, instruments, tools, available data, information, and knowledge relevant to the situation to identify patterns and variances.
- Applies ethical, legal, and privacy guidelines and policies to the collection, maintenance, use, and dissemination of data and information.
- Recognizes the healthcare consumer as the authority on their own health by honoring their care preferences.
- Documents relevant data accurately, timely, and in a manner accessible to the interdisciplinary team.

Additional competencies for the graduate-level prepared registered nurse specializing in nephrology

In addition to the competencies of the nephrology registered nurse, the graduate-level prepared registered nurse specializing in nephrology:

- Evaluates risks and potential risks of kidney disease in individuals, families, and the community.
- Synthesizes the results and information leading to clinical understanding.
- Assesses the effect of interactions among individuals, family, community, and social systems on health and illness.

Additional competencies for the advanced practice registered nurse specializing in nephrology

In addition to the competencies of the registered nurse and graduate-level prepared registered nurse specializing in nephrology, the advanced practice registered nurse specializing in nephrology:

- Initiates diagnostic tests and procedures relevant to the healthcare consumer's current status.
- Uses advanced assessment, knowledge, and skills to maintain, enhance, or improve health conditions.

Standard 2 — Diagnosis

The nephrology registered nurse analyzes the assessment data to determine actual or potential diagnoses, problems, and issues.

Competencies

The nephrology registered nurse:

- Uses assessment data, standardized classification systems, technology, and clinical support tools to articulate actual or potential diagnoses, problems, and issues.
- Verifies the diagnoses, problems, and issues with the individual, family, group, community, population, and interdisciplinary colleagues.
- Identifies actual or potential risks to the healthcare consumer's health and safety or barriers to health, which may include, but are not limited to, interpersonal, systematic, technologic, cultural, or environmental circumstances.
- Prioritizes diagnoses, problems, and issues based on mutually established goals to meet the needs of the healthcare consumer with kidney disease across the health–illness continuum which includes a focus on prevention, slowing progression of kidney disease, management of complications/comorbidities, and palliative care.
- Documents diagnoses, problems, and issues in a manner that facilitates the determination of the expected outcomes and the plan that also meets requirements of dialysis-related licensing and regulatory agencies.

Additional competencies for the graduate-level prepared registered nurse specializing in nephrology

In addition to the competencies of the nephrology registered nurse, the graduate-level prepared registered nurse specializing in nephrology:

- Uses information and communication technologies to analyze diagnostic practice patterns of nurses and other members of the interdisciplinary healthcare team.
- Employs aggregate-level data to articulate current and potential diagnoses, problems, and issues of healthcare consumers and organizational systems.

Additional competencies for the advanced practice registered nurse specializing in nephrology

In addition to the competencies of the registered nurse and graduate-level prepared registered nurse specializing in nephrology, the advanced practice registered nurse specializing in nephrology:

- Formulates a differential diagnosis based on the assessment, history, physical examination, and diagnostic test results.
- Uses the KDOQI (National Kidney Foundation Kidney Disease Outcomes Quality Initiative) chronic kidney disease (CKD) staging classification system and/or the KDIGO (Kidney Disease Improving Global Outcomes) to document specific CKD diagnoses.

Standard 3 Outcomes Identification

The nephrology registered nurse identifies expected outcomes for a plan individualized to the healthcare consumer or the situation.

Competencies

The nephrology registered nurse:

- Engages the healthcare consumer, interdisciplinary team, and others in partnership to identify expected outcomes.
- Formulates culturally sensitive expected outcomes from assessments and diagnoses.
- Uses clinical expertise and current evidence-based practice to identify health risks, benefits, costs, and/or expected trajectory of kidney disease.
- Uses evidence-based tools during review of records for a ready reference of the current professionally accepted clinical practice standards to establish targets for individual clinical outcomes for healthcare consumers undergoing kidney replacement therapy (KRT).
- Collaborates with the healthcare consumer with kidney disease to define expected outcomes integrating the healthcare consumer's culture, values, and socioeconomic and ethical considerations.
- Generates a time frame for attainment of expected outcomes.
- Develops expected outcomes that facilitate coordination of care.

- Modifies expected outcomes based on the evaluation of the status of the healthcare consumer and situation.
- Evaluates the actual outcomes in relation to expected outcomes, safety, and quality standards.
- Documents expected outcomes as measurable goals.

Additional competencies for the graduate-level prepared registered nurse, including the advanced practice registered nurse specializing in nephrology

In addition to the competencies of the nephrology registered nurse, the graduate-level prepared registered nurse or the advanced practice registered nurse specializing in nephrology:

- Integrates scientific evidence and best practices to achieve expected outcomes.
- Defines expected outcomes that incorporate cost and clinical effectiveness and are aligned with the outcomes identified by members of the interdisciplinary team.
- Advocates for outcomes that reflect the healthcare consumer's culture, values, and socioeconomic and ethical considerations.
- Differentiates outcomes that require care process interventions from those that require system-level interventions.

Standard 4 Planning

The nephrology registered nurse develops a plan that prescribes strategies to attain expected, measurable outcomes.

Competencies

The nephrology registered nurse:

- Develops an individualized, holistic, evidence-based plan in partnership with the healthcare consumer and interdisciplinary team that establishes goals and priorities for care while considering healthcare consumer characteristics (e.g., stage of CKD, vascular access type, acuity, transplant status, and/or other unique healthcare consumer needs).
- Incorporates an implementation pathway that describes steps and milestones.

- Establishes the plan priorities with the healthcare consumer and interdisciplinary team.
- Includes evidence-based strategies in the plan to address each of the identified diagnoses, problems, or issues. These strategies may include, but are not limited to:
  - Promotion and restoration of health
  - Prevention of illness, injury, and disease
  - Facilitation of healing
  - Alleviation of suffering
  - Supportive care/palliative care/comfort care
- Identifies cost and economic implications of the plan.
- Advocates for responsible and appropriate use of interventions related to kidney disease to minimize unwarranted or unwanted treatment and/or healthcare consumer suffering.
- Prioritizes elements of the plan based on the assessment of the healthcare consumer's level of risk and safety needs.
- Develops a plan that reflects current standard of care and compliance with current statutes, rules and regulations, and standards.
- Modifies the plan according to the ongoing assessment of the healthcare consumer's response and other outcome indicators.
- Documents the plan using standardized language or recognized terminology.
- Identifies barriers to care, assessment strategies, diagnostic strategies, and therapeutic interventions within the plan that reflect current evidence, including data, research, literature, and expert clinical knowledge.

Additional competencies for the graduate-level prepared registered nurse specializing in nephrology

In addition to the competencies of the nephrology registered nurse, the graduate-level prepared registered nurse specializing in nephrology:

- Designs strategies and tactics to meet the multifaceted and complex needs of healthcare consumers with kidney disease and others.
- Leads the design and development of interdisciplinary processes to address the identified diagnoses, problems, or issues.
- Actively participates in the development and continuous improvement of systems that support the planning process.
- Designs innovative nursing practices.

Additional competencies for the advanced practice registered nurse specializing in nephrology

In addition to the competencies of the registered nurse and graduate-level prepared registered nurse specializing in nephrology, the advanced practice registered nurse specializing in nephrology:

- Integrates assessment strategies, diagnostic strategies, and therapeutic interventions that reflect current evidence-based knowledge and practice.

Standard 5 Implementation

The nephrology registered nurse implements the identified plan.

Competencies

The nephrology registered nurse:

- Partners with the healthcare consumer to implement the plan in a safe, effective, efficient, timely, patient-centered, and equitable manner (IOM, 2010).
- Demonstrates caring behaviors to develop therapeutic relationships.
- Provides culturally congruent, holistic care that focuses on the healthcare consumer and addresses and advocates for the needs of the CKD population across all stages and life spans.
- Integrates critical thinking, patient preferences, and technology solutions to enhance nephrology nursing practice and healthcare consumer outcomes.
- Uses evidence-based interventions and strategies to achieve the mutually identified goals and outcomes specific to the problem or needs.
- Integrates interdisciplinary team partners in implementation of the plan through collaboration and communication across the continuum of care.
- Delegates according to the health, safety, and welfare of the healthcare consumer. Considers the circumstance, person, task, direction, communication, supervision, and evaluation, as well as the regulations of state nurse practice act, institution, and other regulatory entities while maintaining accountability for the care.
- Documents implementation and any modification, including changes or omissions of the identified plan.

Additional competencies for the graduate-level prepared registered nurse specializing in nephrology

In addition to the competencies of the nephrology registered nurse, the graduate-level prepared registered nurse specializing in nephrology:

- Uses systems, organizations, and community resources to lead effective change and implement the plan.
- Applies quality principles while articulating methods, tools, performance measures, and standards as they relate to implementation of the plan.
- Translates evidence into practice.
- Leads interdisciplinary teams to communicate, collaborate, and consult effectively.
- Demonstrates leadership skills that emphasize ethical and critical decision making, effective working relationships, and a systems perspective.
- Serves as a consultant to provide additional insight and potential solutions for patients with kidney disease.
- Uses theory-driven approaches to effect organizational or system change.

Additional competencies for the advanced practice registered nurse specializing in nephrology

In addition to the competencies of the registered nurse and graduate-level prepared registered nurse specializing in nephrology, the advanced practice registered nurse specializing in nephrology:

- Uses prescriptive authority, procedures, referrals, treatments, and therapies in accordance with state and federal laws and regulations.
- Prescribes traditional and integrative evidence-based treatments, therapies, and procedures that are compatible with the healthcare consumer's cultural preferences and norms.
- Prescribes evidence-based pharmacologic agents, procedures, and treatments according to clinical indicators and results of diagnostic and laboratory tests to reduce or eliminate the impact of kidney disease complications.
- Provides clinical consultation for healthcare consumers and professionals related to complex clinical cases to improve care and patient outcomes.

Standard 5a

Coordination of Care

The nephrology registered nurse coordinates care delivery.

Competencies

The nephrology registered nurse:

- Organizes the components of the plan.
- Collaborates with consumers with kidney disease to help manage health care based on mutually agreed-upon outcomes.
- Manages the care of healthcare consumers with kidney disease in order to meet and/or reach mutually agreed-upon goals.
- Engages healthcare consumers in self-care to achieve preferred goals for quality of life.
- Assists healthcare consumers with kidney disease to identify options for care.
- Communicates with healthcare consumers, interdisciplinary team, and community-based resources to effect safe transitions in continuity of care.
- Advocates for the delivery of dignified and holistic care by the interdisciplinary team.
- Documents the coordination of care.

Additional competencies for the graduate-level prepared registered nurse specializing in nephrology

In addition to the competencies of the nephrology registered nurse, the graduate-level prepared registered nurse specializing in nephrology:

- Provides leadership in the coordination of interdisciplinary health care for integrated delivery of healthcare consumer care services to achieve safe, effective, efficient, timely, patient-centered, and equitable care (IOM, 2010).

Additional competencies for the advanced practice registered nurse specializing in nephrology

In addition to the competencies of the registered nurse and graduate-level prepared registered nurse specializing in nephrology, the advanced practice registered nurse specializing in nephrology:

- Manages identified consumer panels or populations.
- Serves as the healthcare consumer's primary and/or specialty care provider and coordinator of healthcare services in accordance with state and federal laws and regulations.
- Synthesizes data and information to prescribe and provide necessary system and community support measures, including modifications of environments.

Standard 5b Health Teaching and Health Promtion

The nephrology registered nurse employs strategies to promote health and a safe environment.

Competencies

The nephrology registered nurse:

- Provides opportunities for the healthcare consumer to identify healthcare promotion, disease prevention, and self-management topics.
- Uses health promotion and health teaching methods in collaboration with the CKD healthcare consumer's values, beliefs, health practices, developmental level, learning needs, readiness, ability to learn, language preference, spirituality, culture, socioeconomic status, stage of CKD, and treatment modality.
- Uses feedback and evaluations from the healthcare consumer to determine the effectiveness of the employed strategies.
- Uses technologies to communicate health promotion and disease prevention information to the healthcare consumer.
- Provides healthcare consumers with information about intended effects and potential adverse effects of the plan of care.
- Engages consumer alliance and advocacy groups in health teaching and health promotion activities for healthcare consumers with CKD.
- Collaborates in the design and provides early chronic kidney disease education in advance of kidney replacement therapy (KRT) that includes information on all modalities, including self-care dialysis and transplantation.
- Educates healthcare consumers with kidney disease and their families on kidney replacement options, palliative/end-of-life care, and rationale for the medical management plan.

- Provides anticipatory guidance to healthcare consumers to promote health and prevent or reduce the risk of negative health outcomes.

Additional competencies for the graduate-level prepared registered nurse, including the advanced practice registered nurse specializing in nephrology

In addition to the competencies of the nephrology registered nurse, the graduate-level prepared registered nurse or the advanced practice registered nurse specializing in nephrology:

- Synthesizes empirical evidence on risk behaviors, gender roles, learning theories, behavioral change theories, motivational theories, translational theories for evidence-based practice, epidemiology, and other related theories and frameworks when designing health education information and programs.
- Evaluates health information resources for applicability, accuracy, readability, and comprehensibility to help healthcare consumers' access quality health information.
- Provides anticipatory guidance to healthcare consumers, families, groups, and communities to promote health and prevent or slow progression of disease and treat comorbidities in persons with CKD stages 1–5 before initiation of KRT.

Standard 6 Evaluation

The nephrology registered nurse evaluates progress toward attainment of goals and outcomes.

Competencies

The nephrology registered nurse:

- Conducts a holistic, systematic, ongoing, and criterion-based evaluation of the goals and outcomes in relation to the structure, processes, and timeline prescribed in the plan of care.
- Collaborates with the healthcare consumer (e.g., individual with chronic kidney disease) and others (e.g., family, healthcare professionals) involved in the care or situation in the evaluation process.
- Collaborates with the healthcare consumer and other stakeholders to reevaluate the appropriateness of the current modality, ability for self-care, referral to

vocational and physical rehabilitation services, and all other criteria mandated by the CMS Conditions for Coverage and Interpretive Guidelines for healthcare consumers undergoing KRT.

- Determines, in partnership with the healthcare consumer and other stakeholders (e.g., interdisciplinary team, family), the person-centeredness, effectiveness, efficiency, safety, timeliness, and equitability (IOM, 2001) of the strategies in relation to the responses to the plan of care and attainment of outcomes. Other defined criteria (e.g., Quality and Safety Education for Nurses [QSEN]) should be considered as appropriate.
- Uses ongoing assessment data to revise the diagnoses, outcomes, plan of care, and implementation of person-centered strategies.
- Shares evaluation data and conclusions with the healthcare consumer and other stakeholders in accordance with federal and state laws and regulations.
- Participates in assessing and ensuring the responsible and appropriate use of interventions and equipment (e.g., dialysis machine), and monitors to promote safety and quality of care and to minimize unwarranted or unwanted treatment and healthcare consumer suffering.
- Documents the results of the evaluation to enhance communication within and across healthcare settings and among healthcare professionals.

Additional competencies for the graduate-level prepared registered nurse, including the advanced practice registered nurse specializing in nephrology

In addition to the competencies of the nephrology registered nurse, the graduate-level prepared registered nurse or the advanced practice registered nurse specializing in nephrology:

- Synthesizes evaluation data from the healthcare consumer, family, interdisciplinary team, community, population and/or institution, networks, and organizations to determine the effectiveness of the plan of care.
- Engages in a systematic evaluation process to revise the plan of care that considers trajectory of illness, life transitions, and treatments based in an effort to achieve quality of care, enhance individual experience of care, and lower healthcare costs.
- Uses the results of the evaluation to make or recommend process, policy, procedure, or protocol revisions as appropriate.

Standards of Professional Performance

The Standards of Professional Performance describe a competent level of behavior in the professional role, including activities related to ethics, culturally congruent practice, communication, collaboration, leadership, education, evidence-based practice and research, quality of practice, professional practice evaluation, resource utilization, and environmental health.

All registered nurses are expected to engage in professional role activities, including leadership, appropriate to their education, experience, and position. Nephrology registered nurses are accountable for their professional actions to themselves, their healthcare consumers, their peers, and ultimately, to society.

Standard 7 Ethics

The nephrology registered nurse practices ethically.

Competencies

The nephrology registered nurse:

- Integrates the *Code of Ethics for Nurses with Interpretive Statements* (ANA, 2015a) to guide nursing practice and articulate the moral foundation of nephrology nursing.
- Practices with compassion and respect for the inherent dignity, worth, and unique attributes of individuals receiving nephrology care whether an individual, family, group, community, or population.
- Recognizes the centrality of the healthcare consumer and family as core members of the healthcare interdisciplinary team.
- Safeguards the privacy and confidentiality of healthcare consumers, others, and their data and information within ethical, legal, and regulatory parameters.
- Advocates for healthcare consumers' rights to be involved in shared decision making about treatment choices for acute and chronic kidney conditions, which include rights for supportive care and rights to informed decision making and self-determination.

- Seeks guidance in situations where the rights of the individual conflict with public health guidelines.
- Endorses the understanding that the primary commitment is to the healthcare consumer regardless of the healthcare setting or situation (e.g., dialysis center protocols).
- Maintains a therapeutic and professional healthcare consumer–nurse relationship with appropriate professional role boundaries.
- Advocates for the rights, health, quality, and safety of the healthcare consumer and others.
- Recognizes that nephrology professionals have frequent encounters with ethical dilemmas due to the nature of the specialty (e.g., appropriateness of kidney replacement therapy, which includes initiation of KRT, withholding treatment and implementation of supportive care, providing a time-limited trial of dialysis, withdrawal from dialysis with hospice care, consumers who discontinue treatment before prescribed time or at prescribed frequency, honoring preexisting advanced directives, or resource allocation).
- Advocates for equitable healthcare consumer care.
- Collaborates with the interdisciplinary team, others, and the public to protect human rights, promote diplomacy, enhance cultural sensitivity, and congruence to reduce health disparities.
- Advances nephrology nursing as a profession through scholarly inquiry (e.g., nursing research and evidence-based practice projects), professional nephrology standards development, and the generation and/or contribution to policy as it relates to ethical issues.
- Contributes to resolving ethical issues/moral distress of healthcare consumers, colleagues, or systems, as evidenced in such activities as participating as members of ethics committees, comprehensive healthcare consumer care conferences, Quality Assessment and Performance Improvement (QAPI) meetings, and development of policies and procedures.
- Articulates nephrology nursing values to maintain personal integrity and the integrity of nephrology professional practice.
- Integrates principles of social justice into nephrology nursing practice and policy-related initiatives.
- Owes the same duties to self as to others, including the responsibility to promote health and safety, preserve wholeness of character and integrity, maintain competence, and continue personal and professional growth.
- Collaborates as necessary to establish, maintain, and improve the ethical

environment of the work setting and conditions of employment that are conducive to safe, quality KRT care.

- Maintains competence through continued personal and professional development.

Additional competencies for the advanced practice registered nurse specializing in nephrology

In addition to the competencies of the nephrology registered nurse, the advanced practice registered nurse specializing in nephrology:

- Engages in collaborative practice with interdisciplinary teams that address ethical risks, benefits, goals, and outcomes.
- Provides information regarding the risks, benefits, goals, and outcomes of healthcare regimens in support of informed decision making by the healthcare consumer that includes the right to agree or refuse aspects of the treatment regimen.
- Collaborates with the interdisciplinary team to provide ethically sound palliative/end-of-life care for patients with CKD.

Standard 8 Culturally Congruent Practice

The nephrology registered nurse practices in a manner that is congruent with cultural diversity and inclusion principles.

Competencies

The nephrology registered nurse:

- Demonstrates knowledge and understanding of the perspectives, traditions, values, practices, and family systems of culturally diverse populations, families, and communities of individuals with acute and chronic kidney conditions across the care continuum.
- Participates in lifelong learning to achieve cultural competence that promotes understanding of cultural preferences, global diversity, and culturally congruent decision making that considers the influence of health traditions (e.g., folk, complementary, and alternative medicine) on health and well-being.
- Creates an inventory of one's own values, beliefs, and cultural heritage.

- Demonstrates cultural humility by recognizing limitations of one's own cultural perspective, values, beliefs, and heritage.
- Removes inherent barriers that may exist, thereby providing better nursing care and demonstrating respect, equity, and empathy in actions and interactions with all healthcare consumers.
- Uses cross-cultural knowledge (e.g., variations in health beliefs, practices, and communication patterns) and cultural sensitivity skills to deliver culturally competent care.
- Identifies the stage of the healthcare consumer's acculturation and accompanying patterns of need and engagement.
- Considers cultural influences (e.g., beliefs, values) on decision making regarding treatment modalities (e.g., dialysis, transplant), supportive care, and end-of-life care.
- Uses skills and available tools that are vetted for the culture, literacy level, and language of the population served.
- Considers the effects and impact of discrimination and oppression on practice within and among vulnerable cultural groups, including lesbian, gay, bisexual, and transgender groups.
- Assesses healthcare consumers' fluency in English (e.g., asks person to repeat back explanation or instructions).
- Engages in cross-cultural communication with appropriate language and nonverbal behaviors, including use of medical interpreters and translators in accordance with healthcare consumers' preferences.
- Identifies the cultural meaning of interactions, terms, and content.
- Advocates for person-centered care that embraces the individual's cultural beliefs and values.
- Promotes equal access to services, diagnostic tests, interventions, health promotion and disease prevention, enrollment in research and/or evidence-based practice projects, education, and other opportunities.
- Educates nurse colleagues and members of interdisciplinary teams regarding racial and ethnic disparities and other biases and prejudices that may exist in healthcare.
- Promotes cross-cultural education that enhances awareness of health professionals and other members of the nephrology care community (e.g., dialysis technicians) regarding cultural and social influences on health and quality care and strategies to improve health outcomes.

Additional competencies for the graduate-level prepared registered nurse specializing in nephrology

In addition to the competencies of the nephrology registered nurse, the graduate-level prepared registered nurse specializing in nephrology:

- Evaluates tools and instruments for validity and reliability in culturally diverse populations.
- Advocates for culturally competent organizations that provide services aimed at meeting the cultural and linguistic needs of healthcare consumers.
- Advances organizational policies, programs, services, and practices that reflect respect, equity, and values for diversity and inclusion.
- Establishes internal and external cross-cultural partnerships with healthcare consumers, key stakeholders, and others.
- Collaborates with other organizational members to develop recruitment and retention strategies that promote diversity of nursing and healthcare workforce (e.g., dialysis technicians).
- Conducts research and/or evidence-based practice projects to improve health care and health outcomes of culturally diverse populations.

Additional competencies for the advanced practice registered nurse specializing in nephrology

In addition to the competencies of the registered nurse and graduate-level prepared registered nurse specializing in nephrology, the advanced practice registered nurse specializing in nephrology:

- Promotes shared decision-making strategies regarding planning, prescribing, and evaluating care processes in situations when the healthcare consumer's cultural preferences and norms may not be congruent with the best available evidence (e.g., research, clinical practice guidelines) and APRN expertise.
- Assumes a leadership role in interdisciplinary teams to identify the cultural and linguistic needs of healthcare consumers with acute and chronic kidney conditions.
- Provides person-centered care recognizing cultural diversity and incorporating cultural and spiritual preferences, values, and beliefs by engaging in shared decision making to mutually establish an acceptable plan of care.

Standard 9 Communication

The nephrology registered nurse communicates effectively in all areas of practice.

Competencies

The nephrology registered nurse:

- Assesses communication format preferences of healthcare consumers, families, and interdisciplinary team members (e.g., physician, advanced practice provider, social worker, renal dietitian, dialysis technician, and pharmacist).
- Assesses one's own communication skills and cross-cultural effectiveness.
- Demonstrates cultural empathy when communicating.
- Assesses communication ability, health literacy, available resources, and preferences of healthcare consumers to help inform the interdisciplinary team and others.
- Uses language assistance for individuals with limited English proficiency to ensure effective communication.
- Incorporates appropriate alternative strategies to communicate effectively with healthcare consumers who have visual, hearing, speech, language, or other communication difficulties.
- Incorporates a culturally sensitive communication style and methods that demonstrate caring, compassion, empathy, respect, authentic presence through active listening, and trust.
- Seeks continuous improvement of one's communication skills and conflict resolution skills.
- Conveys accurate information.
- Maintains communication with the interdisciplinary team and others in care coordination efforts to facilitate safe and quality transitions of care and continuity of care delivery.
- Questions rationale supporting care processes and decisions that don't appear to be in the best interest of the healthcare consumer.
- Discloses observations or concerns related to potential or actual hazards and error in care or practice environment to appropriate level.

- Contributes the nursing perspective in interactions with others and discussions with the interdisciplinary team.
- Demonstrates continuous improvement of communication skills.

Additional competencies for the graduate-level prepared registered nurse, including the advanced practice registered nurse specializing in nephrology

In addition to the competencies of the nephrology registered nurse, the graduate-level prepared registered nurse or the advanced practice registered nurse specializing in nephrology:

- Assumes a leadership role to influence effective cross-cultural communication to promote health in culturally diverse populations with acute and chronic kidney conditions across nephrology care settings.

Standard 10 Collaboration

The nephrology registered nurse collaborates with the healthcare consumer, family, and other key stakeholders in the conduct of nursing practice.

Competencies

The nephrology registered nurse:

- Identifies the areas of expertise and contribution of other professionals and key stakeholders.
- Clearly articulates the nephrology nurse's role and responsibilities within the team.
- Uses the unique and complementary abilities of all members of the team to optimize attainment of desired outcomes.
- Partners with the healthcare consumer and key stakeholders to advocate for and effect change, leading to positive outcomes and quality care.
- Uses appropriate tools and techniques, including information systems and technologies, to facilitate discussion and team functions in a manner that protects dignity, respect, privacy, and confidentiality.
- Promotes engagement through consensus building and conflict management.
- Uses effective group dynamics and strategies to enhance team performance.

- Exhibits dignity and respect when interacting with others and giving and receiving feedback.
- Partners with all stakeholders to create, implement, and evaluate a comprehensive plan.

Additional competencies for the graduate-level prepared registered nurse, including the advanced practice registered nurse specializing in nephrology

In addition to the competencies of the nephrology registered nurse, the graduate-level prepared registered nurse or the advanced practice registered nurse specializing in nephrology:

- Participates in interdisciplinary activities including, but not limited to, education, consultation, management, technologic development, or research to enhance outcomes.
- Provides leadership for establishing, improving, and sustaining collaborative relationships to achieve safe, quality care for healthcare consumers.
- Advances interdisciplinary plan-of-care documentation and communication, rationales for plan-of-care changes, and collaborative discussions to improve healthcare consumer outcomes.

Standard 11 Leadership

The nephrology registered nurse leads within the professional practice setting and the profession.

Competencies

The nephrology registered nurse:

- Contributes to the establishment of an environment that supports and maintains respect, trust, and dignity.
- Encourages innovation in practice and role performance to attain personal and professional plans, goals, and vision.
- Communicates to manage change and address conflict.
- Mentors colleagues for the advancement of nephrology nursing practice and the nursing profession to enhance safe, quality health care.
- Retains accountability for delegated nursing care.
- Contributes to the evolution of the profession through participation in professional organizations.
- Influences policy to promote health.

Additional competencies for the graduate-level prepared registered nurse, including the advanced practice registered nurse specializing in nephrology

In addition to the competencies of the nephrology registered nurse, the graduate-level prepared registered nurse or the advanced practice registered nurse specializing in nephrology:

- Influences decision-making bodies to improve the nephrology nursing practice environment and healthcare consumer outcomes.
- Enhances the effectiveness of the interdisciplinary team.
- Promotes advanced practice nursing in nephrology and role development by interpreting its role for healthcare consumers and policy makers.
- Models expert practice to nurses, other interdisciplinary team members, and healthcare consumers.
- Mentors colleagues in the acquisition of clinical knowledge, skills, abilities, and judgment.

Standard 12 Education

The nephrology registered nurse seeks knowledge and competence that reflects current nursing practice and promotes futuristic thinking.

Competencies

The nephrology registered nurse:

- Identifies learning needs based on nursing knowledge and the various roles the nurse may assume.
- Participates in ongoing educational activities related to nursing and interdisciplinary knowledge bases and professional issues.
- Mentors nurses new to their roles in nephrology for the purpose of ensuring successful enculturation, orientation, and emotional support.
- Demonstrates a commitment to lifelong learning through self-reflection and inquiry to address learning and personal growth.
- Seeks experiences that reflect current practice to maintain and advance knowledge, skills, abilities, and judgment in clinical practice or role performance.
- Acquires knowledge and skills relative to the nephrology role, practice setting, and global or local health situation.
- Participates in formal consultation or informal discussions to address issues in nephrology nursing practice as an application of education and knowledge.
- Identifies modifications or accommodations needed in the delivery of education based on the healthcare consumer and family members' needs.
- Shares educational findings, experiences, and ideas with their peers and the interdisciplinary team.
- Facilitates a work environment supportive of ongoing education of healthcare professionals.
- Supports acculturation of nephrology nurses new to their roles by role modeling, encouraging, and sharing pertinent information relative to optimal care delivery.
- Maintains professional records that provide evidence of individual competence and lifelong learning.

Standard 13 Evidence-Based Practice and Research

The nephrology registered nurse integrates evidence and research findings into practice.

Competencies

The nephrology registered nurse:

- Articulates the values of research and its application relative to the nephrology healthcare setting and practice.
- Identifies questions in the nephrology healthcare setting and nephrology practice that can be answered by nursing research.
- Uses current evidence-based knowledge, including research findings, to guide nephrology practice.
- Incorporates evidence when initiating changes in nephrology nursing practice.
- Participates in the formulation of evidence-based practice through research.
- Promotes ethical principles of research in nephrology practice and the healthcare setting.
- Appraises nursing research for optimal application in nephrology practice and the healthcare setting.
- Shares peer reviewed research findings with colleagues to integrate knowledge into nephrology nursing practice.

Additional competencies for the graduate-level prepared registered nurse, including the advanced practice registered nurse specializing in nephrology

In addition to the competencies of the nephrology registered nurse, the graduate-level prepared registered nurse or the advanced practice registered nurse specializing in nephrology:

- Integrates research-based practice in all settings.
- Uses current healthcare research findings and other evidence to expand knowledge, skills, abilities, and judgment; to enhance role performance; and to increase knowledge of professional issues related to nephrology practice.
- Uses critical thinking skills to connect theory and research to practice.
- Integrates nursing research to improve quality in nursing practice.

- Contributes to nursing knowledge by conducting or synthesizing research and other evidence that discovers, examines, and evaluates current practice, knowledge, theories, criteria, and creative approaches to improve healthcare outcomes for patients with kidney disease.
- Encourages other nurses to develop research skills.
- Performs rigorous critique of evidence derived from databases to generate meaningful evidence for nephrology nursing practice.
- Advocates for the ethical conduct of research and translational scholarship with particular attention to the protection of the healthcare consumer as a research participant.
- Promotes a climate of research and clinical inquiry.
- Disseminates research findings through activities such as knowledge sharing with the interdisciplinary team, presentations, publications, consultation, and journal clubs.

Standard 14 Quality of Practice

The nephrology registered nurse contributes to quality nursing practice.

Competencies

The nephrology registered nurse:

- Ensures that nursing practice is safe, effective, efficient, equitable, timely, and patient-centered (IOM, 1999, 2001).
- Identifies barriers and opportunities to improve healthcare safety, effectiveness, efficiency, equitability, timeliness, and patient-centeredness.
- Recommends strategies to improve nephrology nursing quality.
- Uses creativity and innovation to enhance nephrology nursing care.
- Participates in quality improvement initiatives.
- Collects data to monitor the quality of nephrology nursing practice.
- Contributes in efforts to improve healthcare efficiency.
- Provides critical review and/or evaluation of policies, procedures, and guidelines to improve the quality of healthcare.

- Engages in formal and informal peer review processes.
- Collaborates with the interdisciplinary team to implement and review quality improvement plans and interventions.
- Documents nursing practice in a manner that supports quality and performance improvement initiatives.
- Achieves professional certification, when available.

Additional competencies for the graduate-level prepared registered nurse specializing in nephrology

In addition to the competencies of the nephrology registered nurse, the graduate-level prepared registered nurse specializing in nephrology:

- Analyzes trends in healthcare quality data, including examination of cultural influences and factors.
- Incorporates evidence into nephrology nursing practice to improve outcomes.
- Designs innovations to improve outcomes for patients with kidney disease.
- Provides leadership in the design, implementation, and monitoring of quality improvement activities.
- Designs innovations to effect change in nephrology nursing practice and improve health outcomes.
- Evaluates the practice environment and quality of nephrology nursing care rendered in relation to existing evidence.
- Promotes a practice environment that supports evidence-based healthcare.
- Contributes to nursing and interdisciplinary knowledge through scientific inquiry.
- Encourages professional or specialty certification.
- Engages in development, implementation, evaluation, and/or revision of policies, procedures, and guidelines to improve healthcare quality.
- Uses data and information in system-level decision making.
- Influences the organizational system to improve outcomes.

Additional competencies for the advanced practice registered nurse specializing in nephrology

In addition to the competencies of the registered nurse and graduate-level prepared registered nurse specializing in nephrology, the advanced practice registered nurse specializing in nephrology:

- Engages in comparison evaluations of the effectiveness and efficacy of diagnostic tests, clinical procedures and therapies, and treatment plans, in partnership with healthcare consumers, to optimize health and healthcare quality.
- Designs quality improvement studies, research, initiatives, and programs to improve health outcomes in patients with kidney disease.
- Applies knowledge obtained from advanced preparation, as well as current research and evidence-based information, to clinical decision making at the point of care to achieve optimal health outcomes for patients with kidney disease.
- Uses nephrology nursing standards of practice and available benchmarks as a means to evaluate practice at the individual, departmental, or organizational level.

Standard 15 Professional Practice Evaluation

The nephrology registered nurse evaluates one's own and others' nursing practice.

Competencies

The nephrology registered nurse:

- Engages in self-reflection and self-evaluation of nursing practice on a regular basis, identifying areas of strength as well as areas in which professional growth would be beneficial.
- Adheres to the guidance about professional practice as specified in *Nursing: Scope and Standards of Practice, 3rd Edition*; *Code of Ethics for Nurses with Interpretive Statements*; and *Nephrology Nursing Scope and Standards of Practice, 8th Edition.*
- Ensures that nephrology nursing practice is consistent with regulatory

requirements pertaining to licensure,certification, relevant statutes, rules, and regulations.

- Uses organizational policies and procedures to guide professional practice.
- Influences organizational policies and procedures to promote interdisciplinary evidence-based practice.
- Provides evidence for practice decisions and actions as part of the formal and informal evaluation processes.
- Seeks formal and informal feedback regarding one's own practice from healthcare consumers, peers, colleagues, supervisors, and others.
- Provides peers and others with formal and informal constructive feedback regarding their practice or role performance.
- Takes action to achieve goals identified during the evaluation process.

Standard 16 Resource Utilization

The nephrology registered nurse uses appropriate resources to plan, provide, and sustain evidence-based nursing services that are safe, effective, and fiscally responsible.

Competencies

The nephrology registered nurse:

- Assesses individual healthcare consumer care needs and resources available to achieve desired outcomes for patients with kidney disease.
- Assists the healthcare consumer in factoring costs, risks, and benefits in decisions about care.
- Assists the healthcare consumer in identifying and securing appropriate services to address needs across the healthcare continuum.
- Delegates in accordance with applicable legal and policy parameters.
- Identifies impact of resource allocation on the potential for harm, complexity of the task, and desired outcomes.
- Advocates for resources that enhance nephrology nursing practice.
- Integrates telehealth and mobile health technologies into practice to promote positive interactions between healthcare consumers and nephrology care providers.

- Uses organizational and community resources to implement interdisciplinary plans.
- Addresses discriminatory healthcare practices and the impact on resource allocation.

Additional competencies for the graduate-level prepared registered nurse specializing in nephrology

In addition to the competencies of the nephrology registered nurse, the graduate-level prepared registered nurse specializing in nephrology:

- Designs innovative solutions to use resources effectively and maintain quality.
- Creates evaluation strategies that address cost effectiveness, cost benefit, and efficiency factors associated with nephrology nursing practice.
- Assumes complex and advanced leadership roles to initiate and guide change.

Additional competencies for the advanced practice registered nurse specializing in nephrology

In addition to the competencies of the registered nurse and graduate-level prepared registered nurse specializing in nephrology, the advanced practice registered nurse specializing in nephrology:

- Engages organizational and community resources to formulate and implement interdisciplinary plans.

Standard 17 Environmental Health

The nephrology registered nurse practices in an environmentally safe and healthy manner.

Competencies

The nephrology registered nurse:

- Promotes a safe and healthy workplace and professional practice environment.
- Uses environmental health concepts in practice.
- Assesses the environment to identify risk factors.
- Reduces environmental health risks to self, colleagues, and healthcare consumers.

- Communicates information about environmental health risks and exposure reduction strategies.
- Advocates for the safe, judicious, and appropriate use and disposal of products in health care.
- Incorporates technologies to promote safe practice environments.
- Uses products or treatments consistent with evidence-based practice to reduce environmental threats.
- Participates in developing strategies to promote healthy communities and practice environments.

Additional competencies for the graduate-level prepared registered nurse, including the advanced practice registered nurse specializing in nephrology

In addition to the competencies of the nephrology registered nurse, the graduate-level prepared registered nurse or the advanced practice registered nurse specializing in nephrology:

- Analyzes the impact of social, political, and economic influences on the global environment and human health experience.
- Creates partnerships that promote sustainable global environmental health policies and conditions that focus on prevention of hazards to people and the natural environment (ANA, 2007).

Disclaimer

The forms in Section 3 were created for educational purposes only. They are intended to provide examples of the types of forms that administrators and nephrology registered nurses may want to use to incorporate the *Nephrology Nursing Scope and Standards of Practice* into clinical practice.

The information provided is not intended to establish or replace forms provided by dialysis providers to their facilities. Please check with your manager before implementing any form provided here.

Download these sample forms and examples from https://www.annanurse.org/StandardsForms

Section 3 How to Use the Nephrology Nursing Standards in Practice

The *Nephrology Nursing Scope and Standards of Practice* can be used as educational or professional development materials. This section will serve as a guide to implement the standards into everyday practice. It describes the *who, what, where, when, why*, and *how* of nephrology nursing practice.

The *Nephrology Nursing Scope and Standards of Practice* delineates the professional responsibilities of nephrology nurses engaged in nursing practice regardless of the setting. As such, it can serve as a basis for:

- Quality improvement systems
- Regulatory systems
- Healthcare reimbursement and financing methodologies
- Development and evaluation of nursing service delivery systems and organizational structures
- Certification activities
- Position descriptions and performance appraisals
- Agency policies, procedures, and protocols
- Educational offering goals and objectives
- Establishing the legal standard of care

It is imperative to continue to examine how nephrology standards of professional nursing practice can be disseminated and used more effectively to enhance and promote the quality of nephrology nursing practice. In addition, standards of nephrology nursing practice must be evaluated on an ongoing basis and revised as necessary to reflect current best practices and technology changes. The dynamic nature of the healthcare practice environment and the growing body of nursing research provide both the impetus and the opportunity for nephrology nursing to ensure competent nephrology nursing practice in all settings and to promote ongoing professional development that enhances the quality of nephrology nursing practice.

This section provides the nephrology nurse with examples of how to incorporate the *Nephrology Nursing Scope and Standards of Practice* into clinical practice. There is no limit to its application. These are some examples of situations where referencing the standards enhances nephrology nursing practice.

The following forms are examples and should be modified to meet individual needs of the facility. Please go to www.annanurse.org/StandardsForms to download these documents for personal use. The documents are password protected. When prompted, enter the password *NephrologyNurse* to gain access.

Performance Appraisal Action Plan

A nurse manager can use the *Nephrology Nursing Scope and Standards of Practice* when providing an employee with corrective action. Based on *Standard 1: Assessment*, an appropriate assessment is the collection of comprehensive data pertinent to the healthcare consumer's health and/or the situation. If the nephrology nurse does not document the data, the standard is not met.

Using the *Nephrology Nursing Scope and Standards of Practice*, the manager can review the competencies for *Standard 1: Assessment*. The manager can then document the specific competency in which the nurse is deficient. The standard and related competencies can be used to develop the action plan for correction of the deficiency.

No Name Dialysis Center

Performance Appraisal Action Plan

Employee Name: ______________________ Title: __________

Manager's Name: ______________________ Location/Department: __________

The purpose of this action plan is to identify the behavior(s), performance dimension, or skill(s) that must be improved or developed to meet position expectations. The following strategies outline opportunities for improvement or development. The expectation is that the manager and employee meet periodically (biweekly, monthly) to review progress on action plan components and make necessary changes or revisions as needed.

Dimension Identify area, skill, rated as needs improvement on evaluation	**Action** Include recommendations	**Timeframe/Completion** Deadline
Mary will document the following when completing patient assessments. (Take wording from standard.) Assessment of the Dialysis Patient (Standard 1) • The nephrology registered nurse collects pertinent data and information relative to the healthcare consumer's health or the situation.	• Uses evidence-based assessment techniques, instruments, tools, available data, information, and knowledge relevant to the situation to identify patterns and variances. • Adheres to applicable federal, state, and local regulations for assessment criteria and frequency for healthcare consumers undergoing kidney replacement therapies (KRTs). • Documents relevant data accurately and in a manner accessible to the interprofessional team.	• Completes on 100% of primary care patients over the next 90 days.
2.		
3.		
4.		

Employee Signature: ______________________ Date: __________

Manager Signature: ______________________ Date: __________

Download this sample form from https://www.annanurse.org/StandardsForms

Individual Development Plan (IDP)

Facilities or individual nephrology nurses interested in promoting professional development can apply the standards to the development of an Individual Development Plan (IDP). The IDP can be formulated annually and discussed at an annual review. The *Nephrology Nursing Scope and Standards of Practice* provide an important tool for the nephrology nurse interested in developing short-term and long-term career objectives.

Using *Standard 11: Leadership* and *Standard 12: Education* can assist with the completion of the nurse's IDP. When *Standard 12: Education* is reviewed, the nurse finds two goals that can be completed within a shorter time frame, and describes the activities that will be completed and a method of application of the knowledge gained. *Standard 11: Leadership* is used to begin the process of developing leadership skills. The following IDP tool reflects the nurse's goals:

- Over the next 1 to 2 years, the nurse has a goal of maintaining her or his certification status by attending continuing educational offerings.
- The nurse has a longer term goal of developing leadership competencies and supporting her or his local ANNA chapter in a leadership role.

No Name Dialysis Center

Individual Development Plan (IDP)

Section 1

Name:	Date:
Title & Location:	Employee ID:

Section 2 – Short-range Goals (1–2 years)

Goal	Developmental Activity/Training	How Will Knowledge Be Applied	Completion Date	Status
These goals are taken directly from the competencies section of the Standards for Professional Performance: ***Standard 12: Education.***				
1. Participates in ongoing educational activities related to nursing and interprofessional knowledge bases and professional issues.	1. Will attend two ANNA sponsored conferences within the calendar year.	1. Will present to fellow nephrology nurses information obtained at the conferences.		1. Initiated
2. Seeks experiences that reflect current practice to maintain and advance knowledge, skills, abilities, and judgment in clinical practice or role performance.	2. Volunteer to actively participate on No Name Dialysis Center's Quality Improvement committee.	2. Will assist in improving my clinical practice skills.		2. Active participant

Section 3 – Long-Range Career Goals (2–5+ years)

Goal	Developmental Activity/Training	How Will Knowledge Be Applied	Completion Date	Status
This goal was taken directly from the competencies section of the Standards for Professional Performance: ***Standard 11: Leadership.***				
1. Mentors colleagues for the advancement of nephrology nursing practice and the nursing profession to enhance safe, quality health care.	1. Volunteer at the local ANNA Chapter assisting developing educational conferences for ANNA members.	1. Will assist in developing leadership skills which may be used to mentor colleagues in nephrology nursing.		1. Not initiated at this time

Section 4

Signature:	Date:
Supervisor Signature:	Date:

Download this sample form from https://www.annanurse.org/StandardsForms

Employee Performance Review

A local area administrator is having a difficult time designing a performance review for the nursing staff. Recalling that the *Nephrology Nursing Scope and Standards of Practice* address Standards of Professional Performance, the administrator decides to use these to evaluate the nursing staff.

The administrator collaborates with the facility staff, and they decide that ethics, leadership, communication, collaboration, quality of practice, and environmental health are the areas they will use to evaluate nursing care. Each standard indicates competencies, and these will be incorporated into the performance review form. In addition, the administrator added several key components that were mandated to be included by the corporate office.

No Name Dialysis Center

Employee Performance Review Form

Employee Name	Job Title	Job Date	Review Period
		/ /	/ / thru / /

Rating System
TT = **Top Talent**: Performance exceeds position requirements. Results attained, values clearly demonstrated, and personal contribution is exceptional.
VC = **Valued Contributor**: Performance meets position requirements. Results attained and personal contribution represent the level expected.
NI = **Needs Improvement**: Performance requires improvement in order to meet position requirements. **ACTION PLAN REQUIRED.**

Position-Specific Requirements
Review job description to determine overall rating for job-specific requirements, including essential functions, technical competencies, and job-specific knowledge. Rate results attained for job-specific objectives (**attach applicable job description**):

Ethics *From Standard 7: Ethics* The nephrology registered nurse practices ethically. Please note, (E) = employee's self-evaluation rating, and (M) = manager's rating.	Rating E	Rating M
Integrates the Code of Ethics for Nurses and Interpretive Statements (ANA, 2015a) to guide nursing practice and articulate the moral foundation of nephrology nursing.		
Practices with compassion and respect for the inherent dignity, worth, and unique attributes of individuals receiving nephrology care whether an individual, family, group, community, or population.		
Advocates for healthcare consumers' rights to be involved in shared decision making about treatment choices for acute and chronic kidney conditions, which includes rights for supportive care and rights to informed decision making and self-determination.		
Maintains therapeutic and professional healthcare consumer-nurse relationship with appropriate professional role boundaries.		

Safe Environment *From Standard 17: Environmental Health* The nephrology registered nurse practices in an environmentally safe and healthy manner.	Rating E	Rating M
Promotes a safe and healthy workplace and professional practice environment.		
Advocates for the safe, judicious, and appropriate use and disposal of products in health care.		
Maintains adherence to dress code.		
Reduces environmental health risks to self, colleagues, and healthcare consumers.		

Communication/Collaboration *From Standard 9: Communication and Standard 10: Collaboration* The nephrology registered nurse communicates effectively in a variety of formats and collaborates with healthcare consumer, family, and others in the conduct of nursing practice. Please note, (E) = employee's self-evaluation rating, and (M) = manager's rating.	Rating E	Rating M
Partners with others to effect change and generate positive outcomes through the sharing of knowledge of the healthcare consumer and/or situation.		
Adheres to standards and applicable codes of conduct that govern behavior among peers and colleagues to create a work environment promoting cooperation and respect.		
Maintains communication with other providers to minimize risks associated with transfers and transition of care delivery.		
Communicates effectively in a variety of written, spoken, and technological formats.		
Uses scripts for key customer encounters.		
Follows up on customer requests and issues.		
Looks for opportunities to increase customer satisfaction with service.		
Greets coworkers, visitors, and patients with a smile and "Hello."		
Answers every call with a greeting – "Good Morning/Afternoon" and states facility and name.		
Closes each interaction by asking, "Is there anything else I can do for you?"		

Employee Performance Review Form, continued

Quality of Practice *From Standard 14: Quality of Practice* The nephrology registered nurse contributes to quality nursing practice. Please note: (E) = employee's self-evaluation rating (M) = manager's rating	**Rating** E	M		*Leadership* *From Standard 11: Leadership* The registered nephrology nurse demonstrates leadership in the professional practice setting and the profession. Please note: (E) = employee's self-evaluation rating (M) = manager's rating	**Rating** E	M
Ensures that nursing practice is safe, effective, efficient, equitable, timely, and patient-centered (IOM, 1999, 2001).				Oversees the nursing care given by others while retaining accountability for the quality of care given to the healthcare consumer.		
Provides critical review and/or evaluation of policies, procedures, and guidelines to improve the quality of health care.				Treats others with *respect and dignity*.		
Documents nursing practice in a manner that supports quality and performance improvement initiatives.				Communicates to manage change and address conflict.		
Uses creativity and innovation in nursing practice to enhance nephrology nursing care.				Displays reliability and punctuality.		
				Shares ideas and contributes time to help others (internal and external) of department.		

Performance Highlights/Comments Use this section to record individual pertinent information from the review and comments regarding achievements, accomplishments, strengths, changes in duties, and development areas. Please note: (E) = employee's self-evaluation rating and (M) = manager's rating	**Rating** E M
Job-Specific Objectives: Use this section to record individual goals for the upcoming year that are job-specific. They can be related to change in responsibilities, developing new skills, improving a particular skill, projects, assignments, etc.	

No Name Dialysis Center Employee Requirements		
Department Competencies Met	( ) yes	( ) no
Age-Specific Competencies Met (if applicable)	( ) yes	( ) no
PPD Requirement Met	( ) yes	( ) no
Safety Day Requirement Met	( ) yes	( ) no
Fit Test Requirement Met (if applicable)	( ) yes	( ) no
Attendance Requirement Met	( ) yes	( ) no
HIPAA Confidentiality Requirement Met	( ) yes	( ) no
Dress Code Requirement Met	( ) yes	( ) no
Corporate Compliance Awareness Met	( ) yes	( ) no

Values Grid (use colors)					
Blue = Exceeds Standard/Role Model; **Green**= Consistently Meets Standard; **Red** = Does not Meet Standard/Needs Improvement					
Integrity	**Respect**	**Caring**	**Excellence**	**Commitment**	**Teamwork**
Examples of Blue Values and Red Values in Practice					
Caring – Always takes the time to speak with patients and educate families. (This is blue.) **Commitment** – Often calls out, leaving the staff short of registered nurses on weekends. (This is red.)					

Continues on next page

Employee Performance Review Form*, continued*

Behaviors this individual should KEEP doing:	
Behaviors this individual should STOP doing:	
Behaviors this individual should START doing:	
The next career step(s) for this individual is(are):	

Performance Discussion & Planning

Current BP Rating	
Top Talent	☐
Valued Contributor	☐
Needs Improvement	☐

My personal contribution to No Name Dialysis Center's mission for the coming year is:

1.
2.

Employee's Signature	**Date**	**Supervisor's Signature**	**Date**

For ratings of *Top Talent* and *Needs Improvement*, signature of next level manager is required:

Next Level Signature ______________________________

Date ______________________________

Download this sample form from https://www.annanurse.org/StandardsForms

Policy and Procedure Development

The No Name Dialysis Center has had several episodes with disputes between staff members and patients. On several occasions, the No Name Dialysis Center's administrator had to intervene to provide conflict resolution to resolve patient issues. The No Name Dialysis Center recognizes the need to develop a policy to resolve issues and disputes that arise within the dialysis unit. After reviewing the Standards of Practice, *Standard 17. Environmental Health,* the following competency is noted.

- Promotes a safe and healthy workplace and professional practice environment.
- Assesses the environment to identify risk factors.
- Reduces environmental health risks to self, colleagues, and healthcare consumers.
- Participates in developing strategies to promote healthy communities and practice environments.

Based upon this standard, the following policy was created. While the policy is lengthy, it includes the Standard of Care to be expected within the dialysis facility for each level of aggressive behavior.

No Name Dialysis Center		
Policy and Procedure		
MANUAL TITLE(S)	**Page __ of __**	**Attachments**
MANUAL SECTION	**MANUAL SUBJECT**	
DATE OF ISSUE	**DATE OF REVISION(S)**	**EFFECTIVE DATE**

Purpose

Violence Prevention Program

Policy

- The safety and security of personnel, patients, and visitors is of vital importance. Therefore, acts or threats of physical violence, including intimidation, harassment, or coercion, which occur on No Name Dialysis Center property, will not be tolerated.
- This prohibition against threats and acts of violence applies to all persons involved including, but not limited to, employees, supervisors, physicians, students, contract and temporary personnel, patients, and visitors. Therefore, violations of this policy by any individual on No Name Dialysis Center property are considered misconduct and will lead to disciplinary and/or legal action as appropriate.
- No reprisals will be taken against any employee who reports or experiences workplace violence.
- All No Name Dialysis Center personnel must refrain from engaging in acts of violence and are responsible for maintaining a work environment free from acts or threats of violence.
- Violence Prevention Program Elements:
    - **Conducting an annual assessment** of No Name Dialysis Center property, which includes facility layout, access control, and lighting; crime in the surrounding community; communication equipment; emergency response capabilities
    - **Controlling access to facilities and sensitive areas**
    - **Ensuring adequate security systems,** including card readers, cameras, door locks, windows, physical barriers, and restraint systems are operational and appropriate for the setting
    - **Maintaining effective systems to warn others** of a security danger or to summon assistance (i.e., panic buttons)
    - **Providing adequately trained staff** to provide services and response

Continues on next page

Policy and Procedure – Violence Prevention Program, continued

- **Conducting an Annual Security Opinion Survey** to obtain feedback on services and identify opportunities for improvement
- **Reviewing all incidents** involving security-assisted restraints, disorderly persons, thefts, and assaults. Action plans are developed, implemented, and monitored as appropriate
- **Enforcing Visitor Control** and identification policies
- **Providing Preventing Workplace Violence and Nonviolent Crisis Intervention**/Identification and Management of Aggressive Behavior courses through No Name Dialysis Center corporate office

*** The above bold areas assist in promoting a healthy community from the Standards of Practice.**

Response to Potential Violence

- **When a threat of violence is identified**, a team will be formed to review information and determine the appropriate actions. The team will consist of members from the following departments:
  - Human Resources
  - Nursing
  - Security
  - Risk Management/Legal
  - Public Relations
  - Social Work/Behavioral Health
  - Administration
- The team's duties include, but are not limited to:
  - **Reviewing past incidents** of aggression or violence and identifying the threat level
  - **Referring to the Warning Sign** and Appropriate Response to Aggressive Behavior for guidance
  - **Reviewing the facility's readiness** to respond to issues of aggression or violence
  - **Ensuring adequate security** presence and response is available
  - **Establishing liaison** with local law enforcement and emergency services
  - **Communicating to employees** or others that were or may be involved in an incident involving workplace violence
  - **Assigning all or some** of these tasks to other individuals
- **Managers and supervisors** are responsible for the following:
  - Providing workplace violence prevention training for personnel under their supervision
  - Assisting management response team as necessary

Continues on next page

Policy and Procedure – Violence Prevention Program, continued

- **Reporting Requirements**
  - Employees/Supervisors

  Personnel shall immediately report any acts or threats of violence to the Security Department, their supervisor/manager, or to the Human Resources Department. Employees are additionally required to report the occurrences of each warning sign of violence that they observe (i.e., verbal abuse, aggressive behavior, loitering). No employee will be disciplined or discharged for reporting any threats or acts of violence.

- **Contracted Services**
  - Third parties working on No Name Dialysis Center property shall be informed of Workplace Violence Prevention requirements by Purchasing prior to doing any actual work on facility premises.

- **Postincident Management**
  - Victims of violence will receive immediate physical evaluations, be removed from the worksite, and treated for acute injuries. Additionally, referrals shall be made for appropriate evaluation, treatment, counseling, and assistance, both at the time of the incident and for any follow-up treatment necessary.

- **Record Keeping**
  - Record keeping should be used to provide information for analysis, evaluation of methods of control, severity determinations, identifying training needs, and overall program evaluations. Record keeping includes the following:
    - ✓ **Entry of injury on the OSHA Injury and Illness Log.** Injuries that must be recorded include the following:
      - Loss of consciousness
      - Restriction of work or motions
      - Transfer to another job or termination of employment
      - Medical treatment beyond first aid
    - ✓ **All incidents of abuse, verbal attacks, or aggressive behavior**
    - ✓ **Recording and communicating mechanism** so that staff who provide care for an escalating or potentially aggressive, abusive, or violent patient will be aware of the patient's status and of any problems experienced in the past
    - ✓ **Gathering of information** to identify any past history of violent behavior, incarceration, probation reports, or any other information that assists employees to assess violent status
    - ✓ Workers' Compensation and insurance record
    - ✓ **Environment of Care Committee Minutes** and inspections are kept in accordance with requirements
    - ✓ Training program contents and sign-in sheets of all attendees are maintained

*** The above bold areas assist in preventing/reporting a hostile work environment**

Continues on next page

Policy and Procedure – Violence Prevention Program, continued

Warning Signs and the Appropriate Response to Aggressive Behavior

The following is a guideline for determining the severity of a violent situation and the appropriate response.

Procedure

LOW

These are behaviors that should raise the awareness of the employees and others around the employee, patient, or visitor. It is an indication that a problem is developing and will likely continue without intervention.

Behavioral Examples

Inappropriate behavior
Abusive language
Excessive use of profanity
Argumentative
Lack of cooperation when requests are made
Sexual comments, gestures, or innuendoes
Negative attitude toward the rules
Frequent displays of anger
Emotionally erratic
Veiled threats
Inappropriate use of computers and phone systems

Recommendations

- *Employee*
  Document incident and notify supervisor.
  Supervisor and Human Resources reviews behavioral expectations with employee.
  Consult with Human Resources if behavior continues.
  Coach/counsel employee.
- *Patient*
  Document incident.
  Notify supervisor and security.
  Consider psych consult and 1:1.
- *Visitor*
  Document incident.
  Notify supervisor.
  Notify security.
  Consider visitor restriction or supervised visits.

MEDIUM

These are behaviors that should sound the alarm that the situation is escalating and that without intervention, an incident could occur.

Behavioral Examples

Overt, covert, or indirect threats
Expressed desire to do harm to others

Continues on next page

Policy and Procedure – Violence Prevention Program, continued

Attempts to instigate fights
Open defiance of the rules
Vandalism
Property theft
Belief that others are conspiring against them or prosecuting them
Sexual or violent notes sent to others
Expressed suicidal thoughts or threats
Physical acting out of anger
Comments about weapons or stories of harming others
Severe emotional distress

Recommendations

- *Employee*
  Obtain assistance and guidance from Human Resources, Legal, and Behavioral Health Leadership.
  Document all incidents and assist in the investigation.
  Coach/counsel employee.
- *Patient*
  Document incident.
  Notify supervisor and security.
  Request psych consult and 1:1.
  Consider chemical or physical restraint.
- *Visitor*
  Document incident.
  Notify supervisor and security.
  Notify local law enforcement and consult Legal.

HIGH
These are behaviors that are dangerous and require immediate intervention and assistance.

Behavioral Examples
Clear intent to harm
Physical assault
Intense uncontrollable anger
Overt threats to kill
Showing a weapon
Sabotage with intent to harm others
Suicide attempt

Recommendations

- *Employee*
  Call the local police (911) and security and notify Human Resources for guidance.
  Ensure the safety of all employees, patients, and visitors.
  Document the incident and assist in the investigation.

Continues on next page

Policy and Procedure – Violence Prevention Program, continued

- *Patient*
  Assign 1:1.
  Expedite medical treatment to discharge to behavioral health unit.
  Consider physical restraint and chemical restraint.
- *Visitor*
  Document incident.
  Notify supervisor and security.
  Notify local police department and Legal.

EXTREME
This is a situation where there is ongoing or imminent danger due to physical or armed aggression. Employee should seek safety, call police (911), and stay calm.

Physician order required:	No
Consent required:	No
Who may perform:	RNs, technicians, and other dialysis facility personnel
Who may assist:	RNs, technicians, and other dialysis facility personnel

Current Evidence:
- Promotes a safe and healthy workplace and professional practice environment.
- Uses environmental health concepts in practice.
- Assesses the environment to identify risk factors.
- Reduces environmental health risks to self, colleagues, and healthcare consumers.
- Communicates information about environmental health risks and exposure reduction strategies.
- Advocates for the safe, judicious, and appropriate use and disposal of products in health care
  (*Nephrology Nursing Scope and Standards of Practice, 2017*)

Equipment/Supplies: Not required

Age-specific technical consideration:
Age-specific considerations should be taken into account when type and level of Aggressive Behavior is evaluated.

Continues on next page

Policy and Procedure – Violence Prevention Program, continued

Documentation:
As noted under each level, response to *Warning Signs and the Appropriate Response to Aggressive Behavior*

APPROVED BY:	DATE APPROVED:
SOURCE:	CONCURRED:
DISTRIBUTION: See Distribution list	KEYWORDS:

Download this sample form from https://www.annanurse.org/StandardsForms

Position Description

The nursing staff of the No Name Dialysis Center was asked to develop a position description. The charge nurse had a copy of the *Nephrology Nursing Scope and Standards of Practice,* which they used as a reference. The nursing staff was able to create a position description that included many of the standards within the role statement and job essentials. The role statement includes assessment, diagnosis, outcomes identification, planning, implementation, and evaluation of patient care. The nursing staff also added outcomes identification, ethics, education, evidence-based practice, and research. The nurse manager was impressed with the development of the position description and that the nurses had been able to implement the Scope of Practice within their position description.

No Name Dialysis Center

Job Description

Position Title: Registered Nurse

Reports to: Nurse Manager **Department:** Nursing

Role Statement *

Responsible for assessing, diagnosing, planning, implementing, and evaluating patient care through outcomes identification and evidence-based practice research. As an integral member of the healthcare team, coordinates patient care, and communicates and collaborates extensively with the other members of the healthcare team, patients, and/or patient's family or significant other(s). Maintains and demonstrates high standards of professional ethics.

Job Essentials *

- Performs an assessment of the patient, leading to development, implementation, and evaluation of a plan of care.
- Administers, monitors, and documents therapeutic interventions and regimens.
- Effectively manages rapidly changing situations.
- Participates in clinical decision making.
- Educates patient and family/responsible party regarding disease process, individual care needs, wellness, safety issues, etc.
- Delegates and monitors care rendered by other members of nursing department and healthcare team.
- Demonstrates standard precautions and patient safety principles in practice.
- Participates in orientation, education, and development of healthcare team.
- Identifies and participates in performance improvement activities.
- Maintains professional and departmental level competencies.
- Advocates for the safe, judicious, and appropriate use and disposal of products in health care.

Educational Requirements, Qualifications

- Graduate of an accredited school of nursing.
- Valid RN License in the state of practice. (Refer to the Educational/Regulatory Requirement policy in the Nursing Administrative Manual.)
- Demonstrates knowledge of nursing skills, facility/hospital practices, procedures, and standards.
- Assessment skills, ongoing education.
- Strong communication skills.
- Coordinates and collaborates with a team of care providers.

Job Description

Americans with Disabilities Act (ADA) Requirements:
(Based on a scale of I to V, with V being the highest level)

- Physical Strength – IV
- Manual Dexterity – IV
- Motor Coordination – III
- Form Perception – IV
- Environmental Conditions – I
  - ✓ Environmental hazards – Potential exposure to toxic or caustic chemicals, infectious diseases, radiant energy, electric shock, proximity to moving, mechanical parts, and exposure to combative behavior.
  - ✓ Physical demands – Talking and hearing, vision, stooping, kneeling, crouching, reaching, handling, feeling, fingering.
  - ✓ Machines, equipment, work aids that may be representative but not all-inclusive of those commonly associated with this type of work – electric beds, cardiac monitors, stretchers, wheelchairs, sharp objects (i.e., needles and syringes), oxygen and suction equipment, and other medical equipment, computers, and office equipment.

Download this sample form from https://www.annanurse.org/StandardsForms

Competency Skills Checklist

The mentor of the No Name Transplant Center was asked by the Department Supervisor to develop a skills checklist. The mentor used the *Nephrology Nursing: Scope and Standards of Practice* in the development of the skills checklist. He identified the outcomes for transplant nurses based on the standards of assessment, planning, communication, and collaboration (*Standards 1, 4, 9, and 10*).

Form Guidelines

Purpose

Use this form to outline one or more competencies. List only critical performance criteria to evaluate.

1. State the title[s] of the Competencies or Competency to be evaluated on the top of the form.
2. Print all demographic information as listed.
3. Place a check mark in the box indicating the age requirement(s) related to this competency based on the population served by the department.
4. State the selected Performance Criteria in behavioral terminology in the performance criteria column. (Example: The employee will be able to demonstrate...)
5. Enter the validation method(s), selecting from the alphabetical key on the form.
6. Enter "ME" for Meets Expectation or "NI" for Needs Improvement in the Evaluation Column.
7. Use the Comment Line to indicate follow-up plan if evaluation indicates need for improvement.
8. The validator signs and dates the form in the space provided.

Attach and send form to HR with Performance Evaluation.

No Name Transplant Center

Job/Population Specific Competency Skills Checklist (Clinical)

Name/Title____ **Dept/Unit** __________

Employee ID Number ______________________ **Division**__________________ **Date:** _____/_____/_____

Ages: Neonate (< 30 days); Infant (1 month to 1 year); Toddler (1–3 years); Preschool (3–5 years); School age (6–12 years); Adolescent (13–18 years); Adulthood (18–69 years); Later Adult (> 70 years)

Validation Method:
A = Policy Review
B = Direct Observation
C = Video Review
D = Verbalization
E = Written Exam
F = Case Study Exam
G = Documentation Review
H = Self Learning Module (SLP)
I = Simulated Demonstration
J = Other (specify)
K = N/A

Performance Criteria	Validation Method (May use more than one method)	Evaluation		Comments
Assessment of Kidney Transplant Recipient		Meets Expectations	Needs Improvement	
• Adheres to applicable federal, state, and local regulations for assessment criteria and frequency for healthcare consumers undergoing kidney replacement therapies (KRTs). • Recognizes the importance of the assessment parameters identified by UNOS, WHO (World Health Organization), Healthy People 2020, or other organizations that influence nephrology nursing transplantation practice. • Collects pertinent data, but not limited to demographics, social determinants of health, health disparities, and physical, functional, psychosocial, emotional, cognitive, sexual, cultural, age-related, environmental, spiritual/transpersonal, and economic assessments in a systematic, ongoing process with compassion and respect for the inherent dignity, worth, and unique attributes of every person. • Elicits the healthcare consumer, values, preferences, expressed and unexpressed needs, and knowledge of the healthcare situation. • Engages the healthcare consumer and other interprofessional team members in holistic, culturally sensitive data collection. • Identifies barriers to effective communication based on psychosocial, literacy, financial, and cultural considerations. • Recognizes impact of one's own personal attitudes, values, and beliefs on the assessment process. • Assesses the impact of family dynamics health and wellness. • Uses evidence-based assessment techniques, instruments, tools, available data, information, and knowledge relevant to the situation to identify patterns and variances. • Applies ethical, legal, and privacy guidelines and policies to the collection, maintenance, use, and dissemination of data and information. • Recognizes the healthcare consumer as the authority on their own health by honoring their care preferences. • Documents relevant data accurately and in a manner accessible to the interprofessional team. • Uses appropriate evidenced-based assessment techniques, instruments, and tools.	B. Documents findings in nursing assessment form within 12 hours of admission. F. Prepares and revises nursing care plan that reflects assessment finding.s A. Follows No Name Transplant Center P&P on patient identification and completion of surgical checklist.			

Employee Signature: ____ Date: _____/_____/_____

Validator Signature: ____ Date: _____/_____/_____

Send to HR with Performance Evaluation

Download this sample form from https://www.annanurse.org/StandardsForms

Section 4

References

American Nephrology Nurses Association. (2002). *Advanced practice nurse standards of professional performance.* Pitman, NJ: Author.

American Nephrology Nurses Association. (2004a). *ANNA fact sheet.* Pitman, NJ: Author.

American Nephrology Nurses Association. (2004b). *Discover nephrology nursing.* Pitman, NJ: Author.

American Nephrology Nurses Association. (2004c). *Minimum preparation for entry into nursing practice.* Pitman, NJ: Author.

American Nephrology Nurses Association, Task Force on nurse sensitive outcomes. (2014). *Report to ANNA Board of Directors.*

American Nephrology Nurses Association. (2016). www.annanurse.org

American Nurses Association (ANA). (2007). *ANA Principles of environmental health for nursing practice with implementation strategies.* Silver Spring, MD: nursesbooks.org

American Nurses Association. (2010a). *The nurse's role in ethical and human rights:Protecting and promoting individual worth, dignity, and human rights in practice settings.* Retrieved from http://www.nursingworld.org/MainMenuCategories/EthicsStandards/Ethics-Position-Statements/NursesRole-EthicsHumanRights-PositionStatement.pdf

American Nurses Association. (2010b). *Nursing's social policy statement: The essence of the profession.* Silver Spring, MD: Nursesbooks.org

American Nurses Association. (2014). *Professional role competence position statement.* Retrieved from http://www.nursingworld.org/MainMenuCategories/ThePracticeofProfessionalNursing/NursingStandards/Professional-Role-Competence.html. Not cited. If you elect to address this position statement, please reference the 2014 edition.

American Nurses Association. (2015a). *Code of ethics for nurses with interpretive statements.* Silver Spring. MD: Nursesbooks.org.

American Nurses Association. (2015b). *Nursing: Scope and standards of practice* (3rd ed). Silver Spring, MD: ANA.

American Society for Apheresis. (2010, April 14). *American Society for Apheresis guidelines. Resources for apheresis professionals.* Retrieved from http://www.apheresis.org/?page=guidelines

APRN Consensus Work Group & the National Council of State Boards of Nursing APRN Advisory Committee. (2008, July 7). *APRN Joint Dialogue Group: Consensus model for APRN regulation: Licensure, accreditation, certification and education.* Retrieved from http://www.nursingworld.org/ConsensusModelforAPRN

Bastable, S.B. (2014). *Nurse as educator: Principles of teaching and learning for nursing practice* (4th ed.) Syracuse, NY: Jones and Bartlett.

Benner, P. (1982). From novice to expert. *American Journal of Nursing, 82*(3), 402-407.

Board of Higher Education & Massachusetts Organization of Nurse Executives. (2006). *Creativity and connections: Building the framework for the future of nursing education.* Report from the Invitational Working Session, March 23–24, 2006. Burlington, MA: Massachusetts Organization of Nurse Executives. Retrieved from http://www.mass.edu/currentinit/documents/NursingCreativityAndConnections.pdf

Carper, B.A. (1978). Fundamental patterns of knowing in nursing. *Advances in Nursing Science, 1*(1), 13-24.

Carper, B.A. (1992). Philosophical inquiry in nursing: An application. In J.F. Kikuchi & H. Summons (Eds.), *Philosophic inquiry in nursing* (pp. 71-80). Newbury Park, CA: Sage.

Centers for Medicare and Medicaid Services (CMS) Conditions for Coverage (CfCs) (2008). Retrieved from https://www.cms.gov/Regulations-and-Guidance/Legislation/CFCsAndCoPs/index.html?redirect=/cfcsandcops/16_asc.asp

Centers for Medicare and Medicaid Services (CMS). (2009). CMS manual system: Coverage of kidney disease patient education services. Retrieved from https://www.cms.gov/Regulations-and-Guidance/Guidance/Transmittals/downloads/r1876cp.pdf

Coleman, B.K., & Merrill, J.P. (1952). The artificial kidney. *American Journal of Nursing, 52*(3), 327-329.

Cross, T., Bazron, B., Dennis, K., & Isaacs, M. (1989). Towards a culturally competent system of care (Vol. I). Washington, DC: Georgetown University Child Development Center, CASSP Technical Assistance Center.

Donabedian, A. (2005). Evaluating the quality of medical care. *The Milbank Quarterly, 83*(4), 691-729.

Enworom, C.D., & Tabi, M. (2015). Evaluation of kidney disease education on clinical outcomes and knowledge of self-management behaviors of patients with chronic kidney disease. *Nephrology Nursing Journal, 42*(4), 363-373.

Fawcett, J. (1999). The state of nursing science: Hallmarks of the 20th and 21st centuries. *Nursing Science Quarterly, 9*(3) 59-63.

Fawcett, J. (2012). *The future of nursing: How important is discipline-specific knowledge?* A conversation with Jacqueline Fawcett. Interview by Dr. Janie Butts and Dr. Karen Rich. *Nursing Science Quarterly, 25*(2), 151-154.

Fulton, B.J., & Cameron, E.M. (1989). Perspectives on our beginnings: 1962-1979. *ANNA Journal, 16*(3), 201-203.

Greco, K., & Mahon, S.M. (2015). The kidney in health and disease: Genetics and genomics. In C.S. Counts (Ed.), *Core curriculum for nephrology nursing: Module 2. Physiologic and psychosocial basis for nephrology nursing practice.* (6th ed., p. 4). Pitman NJ: American Nephrology Nurses Association.

Guest, S. (2014). *Handbook of peritoneal dialysis* (2nd ed.). CreateSpace Independent Publishing Platform.

Hain, D.J., & Kear, T.M. (2015) Using evidence-based practice to move beyond doing things the way we have always done them. *Nephrology Nursing Journal, 42*(1), 11-20.

Hoffart, N. (1989). Nephrology nursing 1915-1970: A historical study of the integration of technology and care. *ANNA Journal, 16*(3), 169-178.

Hudson, S., & Prowant, B. (2005). *Nephrology nursing standards of practice and guidelines for care.* Pitman, NJ: American Nephrology Nurses Association.

Institute of Medicine (IOM). (1999). *To err is human: Building a safer system.* Washington, DC: National Academies Press.

Institute of Medicine (IOM). (2001). *Crossing the quality chasm.* Washington, DC: National Academies Press.

Institute of Medicine (IOM). (2010). *The future of nursing: Leading change, advancing health.* Washington, DC: National Academies Press.

Kear, T., & Ulrich, B. (2015). Patient safety culture in nephrology nurse practice settings: Issues, solutions, and best practice. *Nephrology Nursing Journal, 42*(2), 113-122.

Kidney Disease: Improving Global Outcomes (KDIGO). (2009). Clinical practice guidelines for the diagnosis, evaluation, prevention, and treatment of chronic kidney disease – mineral and bone disorder (CKD–MBD). *Kidney International, 76*(Suppl. 113), S 1-130.

Kidney Disease: Improving Global Outcomes (KDIGO) CKD Work Group. (2013). KDIGO 2012 clinical practice guideline for the evaluation and management of chronic kidney disease. *Kidney International Supplements, 2013*(3) 1-150. doi:10.1038/kisup.2012.73

Kim, H.S. (1987). Structuring the nursing knowledge system: A typology of four domains. *Research and Theory for Nursing Practice, 1*(2), 99-110.

Leininger, M. (1988). Leininger's theory of nursing: Cultural care diversity and universality. *Nursing Science Quarterly, 1*(4), 152-160.

Mukamana, D., Dushimiyimana, V., Kayitesi, J., Mudasumbwa, G., Nibagwire, J., Ngendahayo, F., … Rosa, W. (2016). Nephrology nursing in Rwanda: Creating the future through education and organizational partnership. *Nephrology Nursing Journal, 43*(3), 311-315.

National Kidney Foundation (NKF). (2002). K/DOQI clinical practice guidelines for chronic kidney disease: Evaluation, classification and stratification. *American Journal of Kidney Diseases, 39*(Suppl. 1), S1-S266.

Nephrology Nursing Certification Commission. (2005). Retrieved from http://www.nncc-exam.org

Newhouse, R.P. (2010). Clinical guidelines for nursing practice: Are we there yet? *Journal of Nursing Administration, 40*(2), 57-59.

Orem, D.E. (1991). *Nursing: Concepts of practice* (4th ed.). St. Louis, MO: Mosby Year Book Inc.

Parker, J. (1998). Nephrology nursing as a specialty. In J. Parker (Ed.), *Contemporary nephrology nursing* (pp. 3-23). Pitman, NJ: American Nephrology Nurses Association.

Parker, M. (2005). *Nursing theories and nursing practice* (2nd ed.). Philadelphia: F.A. Davis.

Pender, N.J. (1996). *Health promotion in nursing practice* (3rd ed.). Stanford, CT: Appleton and Lange.

Pender, N.J., Murdaugh, C.L., & Parsons, M.A. (2005). *Health promotion in nursing practice* (5th ed.). Upper Saddle River, NJ: Prentice Hall.

Polit, D.F., & Beck, C.T. (2008). Nursing research: *Generating and assessing evidence for nursing practice* (8th ed.). Philadelphia: Lippincott Williams & Wilkins.

Powers, B.A, & Knapp, T.R. (2011). *Dictionary of nursing theory* (4th ed.). New York: Springer.

Reid, K., & Dennison, P. (2011). The clinical nurse leader (CNL): Point-of-care safety clinician. *The Online Journal of Issues in Nursing,* 16(3), Manuscript 4.

Renal Physicians Association and American Society of Nephrology. (2000). *Shared decision-making in the appropriate initiation of and withdrawal from dialysis.* Washington, DC: RPA.

Rettig, R.A. (1991). *Origins of the Medicare kidney disease entitlement: The Social Security amendments of 1972.* National Academies Press. Retrieved from http://www.nap.edu/read/1793/chapter/6

Silva, M.C. (1977). Philosophy, science, theory: Interrelationships and implications for nursing research. *Image – the Journal of Nursing Scholarship,* 9(3), 59-63.

Simmons, L. (2009). Dorothea Orem's self-care theory as related to nursing practice in hemodialysis. *Nephrology Nursing Journal, 36*(4), 419-421.

Smith, K.S. (1994). ANNA's involvement in legislative arena targets all levels of government. In *ANNA: 1969-1994. Celebrating 25 years of service to the nephrology community* (p. 20). Pitman, NJ: American Nephrology Nurses Association.

Smith, M.C. (2014). Disciplinary perspectives linked to middle range theory. In M.J. Smith & P.R. Liehr (Eds.), *Middle range theory for nursing* (3rd ed., pp. 3-14). New York: Springer.

Smith, M.C, & Parker, M.E. (2013). *Nursing theories and nursing practice* (4th ed.). Philadelphia: F.A. Davis Company.

Styles, M.M., Schumann, M.J., Bickford, C.J., & White, K. (2008). *Specialization and credentialing in nursing revisited: Understanding the issues, advancing the profession.* Silver Spring, MD: Nursesbooks.org.

Sue, D.W., Arredondo, P., & McDavis, R.J. (1992). Multicultural counseling competencies and standards: a call to the profession. *Journal of Counseling and Development, 70,* 477-486.

Thomas-Hawkins, C., Denno, M., Currier, H., & Wick, G. (2003). Staff nurses' perceptions of the work environment in free standing hemodialysis facilities. *Nephrology Nursing Journal, 30*(24), 377-386.

Thomas-Hawkins, C., Flynn, L., & Clarke, S. (2008). Relationships between registered nurse staffing, process of nursing care, and nurse-reported patient outcomes in chronic hemodialysis units. *Nephrology Nursing Journal, 35*(2), 123-131.

Ulrich, B.T. (2006). Professional nephrology nursing: The specialty, the community, and the nursing roles. In A. Molzahn (Ed.), *Contemporary nephrology nursing* (2nd ed.). Pitman, NJ: American Nephrology Nurses Association.

Ulrich, B., & Kear, T. (2014a). Patient safety culture in nephrology nurse practice settings: Initial findings. *Nephrology Nursing Journal, 41*(5), 459-475.

Ulrich, B., & Kear, T. (2014b). Patient safety and patient safety culture: Foundations of excellent health care delivery. *Nephrology Nursing Journal, 41*(5), 447-456, 505.

United States Renal Data System (USRDS). (2013). *USRDS 2013 annual data report: Atlas of chronic kidney disease and end-stage renal disease in the United States.* Bethesda, MD: National Institutes of Health, National Institute of Diabetes and Digestive and Kidney Diseases. Retrieved from http://www.cdc.gov/diabetes/pubs/pdf/kidney_Factsheet.pdf

United States Renal Data System (USRDS). (2015a). *USRDS annual data report: Epidemiology of kidney disease in the United States.* National Institutes of Health, National Institute of Diabetes and Digestive and Kidney Diseases, Bethesda, MD, 2015. Retrieved from http://www.usrds.org/2015/view/v2_01.aspx

United States Renal Data System (USRDS). (2015b). USRDS annual data report: Epidemiology of kidney disease in the United States. National Institutes of Health, National Institute of Diabetes and Digestive and Kidney Diseases, Bethesda, MD, 2015. Retrieved from http://www.usrds.org/2015/view/v1_06.aspx#Table_6.2

VanBuskirk, S., (2003). Nephrology nursing shortage and solutions invitational summit: Task forces to follow up on defined projects. *Nephrology Nursing Journal, 30*(4), 410.

Watson, J. (2012). *Human caring science: A theory of nursing* (2nd. ed.). Sudbury, MA: Jones and Bartlett Learning.

Yoder, L.A.G., Xin, W., Norris, K.C., & Yan, G. (2013). Patient care staffing levels and facility characteristics in U.S. hemodialysis facilities. *American Journal of Kidney Diseases, 62*(6), doi:10.1053/j.ajkd.2013.05.007

Section 5

Glossary

Advanced practice registered nurse (APRN)

A nurse who has completed an accredited graduate-level education program preparing her or him for the role of certified nurse practitioner, certified registered nurse anesthetist, certified nurse-midwife, or clinical nurse specialist; has passed a national certification examination that measures the APRN role and population-focused competencies; maintains continued competence as evidenced by recertification; and is licensed to practice as an APRN (adapted from APRN JDG, 2008).

Assessment

A systematic, dynamic process by which the registered nurse, through interaction with the patient, family, groups, communities, populations, and healthcare providers, collects and analyzes data. Assessment may include the following dimensions: physical, psychological, sociocultural, spiritual, cognitive, functional abilities, developmental, economic, and lifestyle.

Autonomy

The capacity of a nurse to determine her or his own actions through independent choice, including demonstration of competence, within the full scope of nursing practice.

Caregiver

A person who provides direct care for another, such as a child, dependent adult, the disabled, or the chronically ill.

Chronic kidney disease (CKD)

A progressive loss in kidney function over a period of months or years. It is divided into stages based on glomerular filtration rate. Defined as kidney damage or GFR less than 60 mL/min/1.73 m^2 for more than 3 months. The KDIGO classification is similar but expands to include cause and albuminuria.

Code of ethics (nursing)

A list of provisions that makes explicit the primary goals, values, and obligations of the nursing profession and expresses its values, duties, and commitments to the society of which it is a part. In the United States, nurses abide by and adhere to the *Guide to the Code of Ethics for Nurses with Interpretive Statements* (ANA, 2015a).

Collaboration
: A professional healthcare partnership grounded in a reciprocal and respectful recognition and acceptance of each partner's unique expertise, power, and sphere of influence and responsibilities; the commonality of goals; the mutual safeguarding of the legitimate interest of each party; and the advantages of such a relationship.

Competency
: An expected and measurable level of nursing performance that integrates knowledge, skills, abilities, and judgment, based on established scientific knowledge and expectations for nursing practice.

Continuity of care
: An interdisciplinary process that includes healthcare consumers, families, and other stakeholders in the development of a coordinated plan of care. This process facilitates the patient's transition between settings and healthcare providers, based on changing needs and available resources.

Delegation
: The transfer of responsibility for the performance of a task from one individual to another while retaining accountability for the outcome. Example: the RN, in delegating a task to an assistive individual, transfers the responsibility for the performance of the task but retains professional accountability for the overall care.

Diagnosis
: A clinical judgment about the healthcare consumer's response to actual or potential health conditions or needs. The diagnosis provides the basis for determination of a plan to achieve expected outcomes. Registered nurses use nursing and medical diagnoses, depending upon educational and clinical preparation and legal authority.

Environment
: The surrounding context, milieu, conditions, or atmosphere in which a registered nurse practices.

Environmental health
: Aspects of human health, including quality of life, that are determined by physical, chemical, biologic, social, and psychological problems in the environment. It also refers to the theory and practice of assessing, correcting, controlling, and preventing those factors in the environment that can potentially adversely affect the health of present and future generations.

ESRD Networks
: The End-Stage Renal Disease Networks were established in 1978 to oversee dialysis centers to ensure patients receive quality care. They collect data, implement quality improvement programs, establish grievance procedures, and provide resources.

Evaluation

The process of determining the progress toward attainment of expected outcomes, including the effectiveness of care.

Expected outcomes

End results that are measurable, desirable, and observable, and translate into observable behaviors.

Evidence-based practice

A scholarly and systematic problem-solving paradigm that results in the delivery of high quality health care.

Family

Family of origin or significant others as identified by the healthcare consumer.

Graduate-level prepared registered nurse

A registered nurse prepared at the master's or doctoral educational level who has advanced knowledge, skills, abilities, and judgment; functions in an advanced level as designated by elements of his or her position; and is not required to have additional regulatory oversight.

Health

An experience that is often expressed in terms of wellness and illness, and may occur in the presence or absence of disease or injury.

Healthcare consumer

The person, client, family, group, community, or population that is the focus of attention and to whom the registered nurse is providing services as sanctioned by the state regulatory bodies.

Healthcare providers

Individuals with special expertise who provide healthcare services or assistance to patients. They may include nurses, physicians, psychologists, social workers, nutritionists/dietitians, and various therapists.

Illness

The subjective experience of discomfort.

Implementation

Activities such as teaching, monitoring, providing, counseling, delegating, and coordinating.

Information

Data that is interpreted, organized, or structured.

Interdisciplinary
: Reliant on the overlapping knowledge, skills, and abilities of each professional team member. Consists of, at a minimum, the patient or the patient's designee (if the patient chooses), a registered nurse, a physician treating the patient for ESRD (APRN or PA may substitute for physician), a social worker, and a dietitian.

Interprofessional
: Reliant on the overlapping knowledge, skills, and abilities of each professional team member. Outcomes are enhanced by the team vs. individual members.

Kidney Disease Improving Global Outcomes (KDIGO)
: An international foundation administered by the National Kidney Foundation (U.S.) that aims to foster collaboration in the study of kidney diseases and the dissemination of the best treatment practices through the publication of clinical guidelines

Kidney Disease Outcomes Quality Initiative (KDOQI)
: National Kidney Foundation's Guidelines – Kidney Disease Outcomes Quality Initiative.

KRT
: Kidney replacement therapies; new term being used in place of *renal replacement therapies (RRT)*. These terms identify all therapies used to treat kidney disease, which include dialysis, transplantation, and palliative care.

Medical home
: Care that uses primary care providers to ensure the delivery of coordinated, comprehensive care.

Medicare ESRD Program
: The Medicare ESRD Program was established in 1972. The program provides benefits to patients with kidney disease who are entitled to Social Security benefits.

Nephrology nursing
: Nephrology nursing is a specialty practice addressing the protection, promotion, and optimization of health abilities, prevention of illness and injury, facilitation of healing, alleviation of suffering through the diagnosis and treatment of human response, and advocacy in the care of individuals, families, groups, communities, and populations affected by kidney disease.

Nurse Practice Acts (NPS)
: Each state requires a nurse to be licensed to practice in that state. Nurses are responsible for understanding the NPA in the state(s) where they practice.

Nursing

The protection, promotion, and optimization of health and abilities; prevention of illness and injury; facilitation of healing; alleviation of suffering through the diagnosis and treatment of human response; and advocacy in the care of individuals, families, groups, communities, and populations.

Nursing practice

The collective professional activities of nurses that is characterized by the interrelations of human responses, theory application, nursing actions, and outcomes.

Nursing process

A critical thinking model used by nurses that is characterized by the integration of the singular, concurrent actions of these six components: assessment, diagnosis, identification of outcomes, planning, implementation, and evaluation.

Palliative Ccare

Comprehensive, interdisciplinary care of patients and families facing a chronic or terminal illness focusing primarily on comfort and support. It affirms life and regards dying as a normal process. It neither hastens nor postpones death. It includes relief from pain and other distressing physical symptoms and advance care planning. It integrates the psychological and spiritual aspects of patient care and offers a support system to help the family cope during the patient's illness and in their own bereavement. The goals of palliative care are relief of suffering and maximization of quality of life (RPA/ASN Position on Quality Care at the End of Life, 2002).

Patient

See healthcare consumer.

Peer review

A collegial, systematic, and periodic process by which registered nurses are held accountable for practice and which fosters the refinement of one's knowledge, skills, and decision making at all levels and in all areas of practice.

Plan

A comprehensive outline of the components that need to be addressed to attain expected outcomes.

Quality

The degree to which health services for patients, families, groups, communities, or populations increase the likelihood of desired outcomes and are consistent with current professional knowledge.

Registered nurse (RN)

An individual registered or licensed by a state, commonwealth, territory, government, or other regulatory body to practice as a registered nurse.

Scope of nephrology nursing practice

The description of the who, what, where, when, why, and how of nephrology nursing practice. When considered in conjunction with the *Nephrology Nursing Standards of Professional Practice* and the *ANA Code of Ethics for Nurses*, comprehensively describes the competent level of nephrology nursing.

Scope of nursing practice

The description of the who, what, where, when, why, and how of nursing practice that addresses the range of nursing practice activities common to all registered nurses. When considered in conjunction with the *Standards of Professional Nursing Practice* and the *Code of Ethics for Nurses*, comprehensively describes the competent level of nursing common to all registered nurses.

Standards

Authoritative statements defined and promoted by the profession by which the quality of practice, service, or education can be evaluated.

Standards of nephrology practice

Describe a competent level of nephrology nursing care as demonstrated by the nursing process.

Standards of professional nursing practice

Authoritative statements of the duties that all registered nurses, regardless of role, population, or specialty, are expected to perform competently.

Standards of professional performance

Describe a competent level of behavior in the professional role.

Supportive care

See Palliative care

Section 6

Appendices

Position Statements

A. Delegation of Nursing Care Activities

B. Advanced Practice in Nephrology Nursing

C. Certification in Nephrology Nursing

D. ANNA Health Policy Statement

ANNA Endorsements

E. Principles and Elements of a Healthful Practice/Work Environment

Download these documents from
https://www.annanurse.org/advocacy/resources-and-tools/position-statements

Appendix A Delegation of Nursing Care Activities (page 1 of 3)

ANNA Learning Leading Connecting
American Nephrology Nurses Association

Position Statement

Delegation of Nursing Care Activities

The American Nephrology Nurses Association (ANNA) believes every patient has the right to professional nursing care that encompasses all aspects of the nursing process and meets or exceeds the *ANNA Nephrology Nursing Scope and Standards of Practice* and Centers for Medicare and Medicaid Services (CMS) Conditions for Coverage. The practice of each nurse must comply with the scope of practice, regulations/laws, and licensure requirements of the state in which they are employed. The care of each patient includes, but is not limited to, assessment of patient needs, the development of a comprehensive interdisciplinary patient specific plan of care, implementation of nursing interventions, and the monitoring and evaluation of patient outcomes. The ultimate goal of the nursing process is to effect positive patient outcomes in the most cost effective way. ANNA recognizes that achievement of favorable patient outcomes is a collaborative effort between all members of the interdisciplinary team.

It is the position of ANNA that:

- The RN uses critical thinking and professional judgment when following the Five **Rights** of Delegation, to be sure that the delegation or assignment is:
  1. The **right** task
  2. Under the **right** circumstances
  3. To the **right** person
  4. With the **right** directions and communications; and
  5. Under the **right** supervision and evaluation
     (Joint Statement on Delegation American Nurses Association (ANA) and the National Council of State Boards of Nursing (NCSBN))

- The registered nurse must never delegate a nursing care activity that requires:
  a. The knowledge and expertise derived from completion of a nursing education program and the specialized skill, judgment and decision-making of a registered nurse.
  b. Complex observation, critical decision-making, exercise of nursing judgment, or repeated nursing assessments.
  c. An understanding of the core nephrology nursing principles necessary to recognize and manage real or potential complications that may result in an adverse outcome to the health and safety of the patient.
- The registered nurse is accountable for the:
  a. Safety of the patient
  b. Nursing process
  c. Patient Assessment
  d. Delegation of nursing tasks appropriate to the delegates' documented knowledge, skills, cultural competence, experience, and abilities, within the scope of practice, and the licensure requirements in effect in the state in which the nurse is employed.

ANNA National Office
East Holly Avenue, Box 56 I Pitman, NJ 08071-0056
888-600-ANNA (2662) I 856-256-2320 I Fax: 856-589-7463 I anna@annanurse.org I www.annanurse.org

Download this position statement from
https://www.annanurse.org/advocacy/resources-and-tools/position-statements

Appendix A Delegation of Nursing Care Activities (page 2 of 3)

- Delegation of nursing care activities to licensed practical/vocational nurses (LPN/LVNs) and/or certified dialysis patient care technicians (PCT)/ Certified Clinical Hemodialysis Technician (CCHT) shall comply with the following criteria:

  a. The registered nurse must complete an assessment of the patient's nursing care needs prior to delegating any nursing intervention.
  b. The registered nurse shall be accountable and responsible for all delegated nursing care activities or interventions, and she/he must remain present in the patient care area for ongoing monitoring and evaluation of the patient's response to the therapy.
  c. The patient care activities must be within the licensure and/or certification requirements for the LPN/LVN or PCT/CCHT, practice setting, scope of practice, and the licensure requirements in effect in the state in which the nurse is employed. Additional specific facility/agency policies and procedures related to delegation may also apply.
  d. The registered nurse shall have either instructed the LPN/LVN or PCT/CCHT in the delegated nursing care activity or verified the individual's competency to perform the activity. Persons to whom tasks are delegated should have the opportunity to ask questions and/or request clarification of expectations.
  e. Clinical competency of these individual's will be documented and available, and verified at least annually.
  f. Administration of medication is a nursing responsibility requiring knowledge of the indications, pharmacokinetic action, potential adverse reactions, correct dosage and contraindications, and, in general, is beyond the scope of practice of a PCT/CCHT. Administration of medications by PCT/CCHT's shall be limited to those medications considered part of the routine hemodialysis treatment, that is, normal saline and heparin via the extracorporeal circuit, intradermal lidocaine, and oxygen by nasal cannula, as allowed by the scope of practice, and licensure requirements in effect in the state in which the nurse or PCT/CCHT is employed.
  g. Administration of any blood products and/or intravenous medications by infusion is a nursing responsibility and beyond the scope of practice of the PCT/CCHT.

- The registered nurse is legally accountable and clinically responsible for the complete documentation of the entire nursing process. When certain aspects of the nursing care activities or interventions are delegated to other personnel, the registered nurse retains the legal accountability and clinical responsibility for these activities.
- Registered Nurses are accountable and responsible for the assignment or delegation of nursing activities. Such assignments or delegation must be consistent with state practice acts, organizational policy and nursing standards of practice.

Background and Rationale

The relationship between the registered nurse and the patient constitutes a legal and binding contract. The existence of this contract has been established through case law.

ANNA recognizes potential contributions to the care of nephrology patients by LPN/LVNs and PCT/CCHT's. The scope of practice of the registered nurse in the state where the nurse is employed may limit delegation of nursing care activities or interventions to these licensed and certified personnel.

ANNA National Office
East Holly Avenue, Box 56 I Pitman, NJ 08071-0056
888-600-ANNA (2662) I 856-256-2320 I Fax: 856-589-7463 I anna@annanurse.org I www.annanurse.org

Appendix A Delegation of Nursing Care Activities (page 3 of 3)

References

American Nurses Association (ANA). (2015). *Code of ethics for nurses with interpretive statements.* Washington, DC: http://www.nursingworld.org/DocumentVault/Ethics_1/Code-of-Ethics-for-Nurses.html
.

https://www.ncsbn.org/Delegation_joint_statement_NCSBN-ANA.pdf

Centers for Medicare & Medicaid Services (CMS). (2008). *Medicare and Medicaid Programs; Conditions for Coverage for End-Stage Renal Disease Facilities; Final Rule.* Final rule displayed at: http://www.cms.gov/Regulations-and-Guidance/Legislation/CFCsAndCoPs/downloads/ESRDfinalrule0415.pdf.

Adopted by the ANNA Board of Directors in February 1986
Revised and/or reaffirmed biennially from 1987-2012
Most recently revised: December 2015

ANNA Position Statements are reviewed and reaffirmed biennially.

ANNA National Office
East Holly Avenue, Box 56 I Pitman, NJ 08071-0056
888-600-ANNA (2662) I 856-256-2320 I Fax: 856-589-7463 I anna@annanurse.org I www.annanurse.org

Appendix B Advanced Practice in Nephrology Nursing (page 1 of 3)

ANNA Learning Leading Connecting
American Nephrology Nurses Association

Position Statement

Advanced Practice in Nephrology Nursing

The present health care environment mandates increased access to high quality, cost-effective, patient and family focused care. Trends in the incidence and prevalence of chronic kidney disease (CKD) indicate that this patient population will continue to grow. This growth will be accompanied by an increased need for qualified health care providers who have the knowledge and skills to manage, provide, and coordinate the care of this complex patient population. Advance Practice Registered Nurses (APRNs) in nephrology nursing are qualified providers to meet the needs of this patient population.

It is the position of the American Nephrology Nurses Association (ANNA) that:

- The APRN in nephrology, transplantation and related therapies, by virtue of education, training, and certification, as well as documented competencies, is able to provide safe, competent, high-quality care in a cost-effective manner. In addition, the APRN focuses on promoting the health and well-being of patients and on preventing disease and/or its subsequent complications along the entire continuum of kidney dysfunction. The APRN may provide and coordinate the care of patients with kidney disease in the acute, chronic, and primary care settings and across all treatment modalities. The APRN is an integral member of the health care team and works collaboratively with other health care professionals to assure the highest standard of quality care.

- The clinical role is central to the APRN. Nurses with graduate degrees may hold a variety of positions including, but not limited to, management, research, education, case management, and quality management. The advanced practice nurse works collaboratively with these professionals to provide quality care.

- Consistent with ANA's Nursing's Social Policy Statement and Consensus Model for APRN Regulation: Licensure, Accreditation, Certification & Education (APRN Consensus Work Group, 2008), the minimum requirements for an APRN with specialization in nephrology are graduate level preparation and initial certification in an APRN role in one population focus, including family/individual across the lifespan, adult-gerontology, neonatal, pediatrics, women's health/gender related, and/or psychiatric-mental health. Certification of the APRN as a clinical nurse specialist or nurse practitioner is a method to recognize competence by the profession. Certification at the advanced practice level requires a graduate degree from an accredited program that provides both the necessary didactic and clinical experiences in the area of certification. The APRN in nephrology nursing refers exclusively to those caring for patients in the nurse practitioner or clinical specialist role with prescriptive and autonomous authority as defined by each state's nurse practice act. Additional certification as a Certified Nephrology Nurse (CNN) or Certified Nephrology Nurse - Nurse Practitioner (CNN-NP) is preferred.

- The scope of practice of the APRN should allow maximum utilization of their training and skill set including autonomous practice and full prescriptive authority with support of this practice within each state's nurse practice act. APRN regulations should be revised as necessary to support portability within states. The APRN should be recognized by insurance panels for direct reimbursement.

ANNA National Office
East Holly Avenue, Box 56 I Pitman, NJ 08071-0056
888-600-ANNA (2662) I 856-256-2320 I Fax: 856-589-7463 I anna@annanurse.org I www.annanurse.org

Download this position statement from
https://www.annanurse.org/advocacy/resources-and-tools/position-statements

Appendix B Advanced Practice in Nephrology Nursing (page 2 of 3)

- The APRN should be included in care models/projects, e.g. End Stage Renal Disease Seamless Care Organizations (ESCOs), and/or Disease Management Programs, to assist in the development and facilitation of standards of care to improve kidney care.

Skill sets of the APRN in nephrology include the ability to:

a. Independently assess, conceptualize, diagnose and coordinate care for complex health problems;
b. Assess the health care needs of individuals, families, groups and communities across the health care continuum;
c. Use the nursing process to diagnose, plan, implement, and manage care as well as to evaluate the outcomes of that care;
d. Provide expert nursing care to individuals with varying degrees of kidney impairment;
e. Assist patients and families with modality choices (including hemodialysis, peritoneal dialysis, transplant, and conservative management);
f. Prescribe, administer, and evaluate pharmacologic and non-pharmacologic therapeutic treatment regimens;
g. Focus on care that promotes health, prevents kidney disease, presents and/or manages the complications of acute and chronic disease and prevents disability;
h. Support the palliative care and end-of-life needs of patients and their families;
i. Manage acute and chronic kidney disease in a variety of health care settings;
j. Explore, test, and advance scientific theories upon which nursing practice is based;
k. Provide leadership within the area of nephrology through consultation, clinical practice, education, and research;
l. Contribute to the generation of the knowledge base for nursing and specifically nephrology nursing through research, publications, presentations, and participation in the development of standards and clinical practice guidelines;
m. Provide leadership for practice changes through advocacy and legislative activities;
n. Provide leadership for nephrology nursing to be an integral part of disease management proposals, quality improvement measures and outcome management activities; and
o. Contribute to the advancement of the profession as a whole.

Reference

APRN Joint Dialogue Group. (2008). *Consensus model for APRN regulation: Licensure, accreditation, certification and education.* Retrieved from http://www.nursingworld.org/ConsensusModelforAPRN.

Suggested Readings

Fowler, M.D.M. (2008). *Guide to the code of ethics for nurses: Interpretation and application.* Washington, DC: American Nurses Association.

Gomez, N. (2011). *Nephrology nursing scope and standards of practice* (7th ed). Pitman, NJ: American Nephrology Nurses' Association.

National Governors Association. (2012). *The role of the nurse practitioner in meeting the demand for primary care.*

Pearson Report. (2009, February). *The American Journal of Nurse Practitioners, 13*(2). Retrieved July 7, 2013 from http://www.npwh.org/files/public/PEARSON.pdf.

ANNA National Office
East Holly Avenue, Box 56 I Pitman, NJ 08071-0056
888-600-ANNA (2662) I 856-256-2320 I Fax: 856-589-7463 I anna@annanurse.org I www.annanurse.org

Appendix B Advanced Practice in Nephrology Nursing (page 3 of 3)

Advanced practice nurse job summary. Retrieved July 7, 2013 from www.annanurse.org/download/reference/practice/apnJobDescription.doc.

Institute of Medicine. (2010). *The future of nursing: Leading change, advancing health.* Retrieved July 14, 2013 from http://www.iom.edu/Reports/2010/The-future-of-nursing-leading-change-advancing-health.aspx.

Adopted by the ANNA Board of Directors
Revised and/or reaffirmed biennially from 1997-2013
Most recently revised: December 2015

ANNA Position Statements are reviewed and reaffirmed biennially.

ANNA National Office
East Holly Avenue, Box 56 I Pitman, NJ 08071-0056
888-600-ANNA (2662) I 856-256-2320 I Fax: 856-589-7463 I anna@annanurse.org I www.annanurse.org

Appendix C Certification in Nephrology Nursing (page 1 of 3)

ANNA Learning Leading Connecting
American Nephrology Nurses Association

Position Statement

Certification in Nephrology Nursing

Certification is defined by the American Board of Nursing Specialties (ABNS) as "the formal recognition of specialized knowledge, skills, and experience demonstrated by achievement of standards identified by a nursing specialty to promote optimal health outcomes" (ABNS, 2012). The American Nurses Association (ANA) defines certification as "the process by which a nongovernmental agency or an association grants recognition to an individual who has met certain predetermined qualifications. Certification can be used for entry into practice, validation of competence, recognition of excellence, and/or regulation. It can be mandatory or voluntary. Certification validates an individual's knowledge and skills in a defined role and clinical area of practice, based on predetermined standards" (ANA, 2012).

The American Nephrology Nurses Association (ANNA), in addition to ANA, recognizes nephrology nursing practice as a distinct nursing specialty.

It is the position of ANNA that:

- Certification is an essential component to the internal management of specialty nursing practice.
- Certification assists in protecting the public from unsafe and incompetent caregivers.
- The association will recognize and endorse certification credentials in which:
  - The examination is based on periodic practice analysis surveys.
  - The credentialing body submits to an external peer review process, ensuring the validity and integrity of the certification credential.
- Nursing practice has many levels of experience: novice, advanced beginner, competent, proficient, and expert (Benner, 1984).
- Certification is encouraged for all levels of nephrology nursing practice.

Background and Rationale

ANNA identified certification as an essential component of the model of nephrology nursing specialty practice (Jordan, 1993). ANNA recognized the need for autonomy of the certification body and wrote its first position statement on this topic in 2001. As the professional association for the specialty, ANNA has an inherent interest in the certification of nurses practicing in the specialty. Parker (1998) identified the conferring of a standardized credential as an important means of internal management of specialty nursing practice.

As early as 1979, the ANA acknowledged that the main objective of certification in nursing is to assure that the public receives quality-nursing care and is safe from incompetent caregivers. Other benefits of certification may include quality care and patient satisfaction, professional recognition, financial compensation, career advancement, staff retention, personal growth, self-confidence and professional autonomy (Cary, 2001). Certified nurses also report empowerment and enhanced collaboration with other healthcare professionals (Wade, 2009). A study by Kendall-Gallagher et al. (2011) reinforces the association between nursing expertise and patient outcomes. Wade (2009) describes that the expertise associated with certification improves the quality of patient care.

ANNA National Office
East Holly Avenue, Box 56 I Pitman, NJ 08071-0056
888-600-ANNA (2662) I 856-256-2320 I Fax: 856-589-7463 I anna@annanurse.org I www.annanurse.org

Download this position statement from
https://www.annanurse.org/advocacy/resources-and-tools/position-statements

Appendix C Certification in Nephrology Nursing (page 2 of 3)

Page 2
Certification in Nephrology Nursing

The need to protect the public demands the credential reflect actual practice while also allowing the public to infer the qualifications of the credentialed provider (Joel, 1989; Styles, 1989). Basing a test's blueprint on periodic assessment of current practice via practice analysis surveys provides confidence that the examination reflects up-to-date practice. Practice analysis supported examinations may test at any level of nursing practice.

The integrity, validity, and reliability of the examination and the entire credentialing process is strengthened by external peer review to set standards for test construction and validity, test administration, candidate eligibility, scoring and recertification (ABNS, 1997). The Accreditation Board for Specialty Nursing Certification (ABSNC), formerly the ABNS Accreditation Council, is the only accrediting body specifically for nursing certification. ABSNC accreditation is a peer-review mechanism that allows nursing certification organizations to obtain accreditation by demonstrating compliance with the highest quality standards available in the industry (ABSNC, 2012).

References

Accreditation Board for Specialty Nursing Certification. (2012). *American Board of Accreditation Standards.* Aurora, OH: Author.

American Board of Nursing Specialties. (1997). *Application for approval: Standards, rationale, criteria, required documentation.* Washington, DC: Author.

American Board of Nursing Specialties. (2012). *About us.* Aurora, OH: Author. Retrieved from www.nursingcertification.org.

American Nephrology Nurses' Association. (2001) *Position statement on the autonomy of the NNCC.* Pitman, NJ: Author.

American Nurses Association. (1979). *The study of credentialing in nursing: A new approach.* Kansas City, MO: Author.

American Nurses Association, (2012). *Certification general testing and renewal handbook.* Silver Spring, MD: Author. Retrieved from http://www.nursecredentialing.org/CertificationHandbook.aspx.

Benner, P. (1984). *From novice to expert: Excellence and power in clinical nursing.* Menlo Park, CA: Addison Wesley.

Cary, A.H. (2001). Certified registered nurses: Results of the study of the certified workforce. *American Journal of Nursing, 101*(1), 44-51.

Joel, L. (1989). In search of a rational future for certification. *American Nurse, 21*(10).

Jordan, P.J. (1993). *Nephrology nursing: A guide to professional development.* Pitman, NJ: American Nephrology Nurses' Association.

Kendall-Gallagher, D., Aiken, L. H., Sloane, D. M., & Cimotti, J. P. (2011). Nurse specialty certification, inpatient mortality, and failure to rescue. *Journal of Nursing Scholarship, 43,* 188-194.

Parker, J. (1998) Nephrology nursing as a specialty. In J. Parker (Ed.), *Contemporary nephrology nursing.* Pitman, NJ: American Nephrology Nurses' Association.

ANNA National Office
East Holly Avenue, Box 56 I Pitman, NJ 08071-0056
888-600-ANNA (2662) I 856-256-2320 I Fax: 856-589-7463 I anna@annanurse.org I www.annanurse.org

Appendix C Certification in Nephrology Nursing (page 3 of 3)

Styles, M. (1989). *On specialization in nursing: Towards a new empowerment.* Kansas City, MO: American Nurses Foundation, Inc.

Wade, C. H. (2009). Perceived effects of specialty nurse certification. A review of literature. *AORN Journal*, *89*(1), 184-192.

Adopted by the American Nephrology Nurses' Association
Board of Directors
March 2003
Revised and/or reaffirmed biennially 2003-2013
Reaffirmed: December 2015

ANNA Position Statements are reviewed and reaffirmed biennially.

ANNA National Office
East Holly Avenue, Box 56 I Pitman, NJ 08071-0056
888-600-ANNA (2662) I 856-256-2320 I Fax: 856-589-7463 I anna@annanurse.org I www.annanurse.org

Appendix D ANNA Health Policy Statement (page 1 of 6)

ANNA Learning Leading Connecting
American Nephrology Nurses Association

HEALTH POLICY STATEMENT

PREAMBLE

The American Nephrology Nurses Association (ANNA) is a national organization of registered nurses practicing in nephrology, which includes but is not limited to chronic kidney disease (CKD), hemodialysis, peritoneal dialysis, transplantation, and continuous renal replacement therapies. ANNA members are involved in the supervision and delivery of care to children and adults who have or are at risk of kidney disease. ANNA supports the interdisciplinary approach to health care and believes that registered nurses must be major participants in the planning, delivery, and evaluation of that care.

As a professional organization, ANNA has the obligation to set and update standards of patient care, educate practitioners, stimulate research and disseminate findings, promote interdisciplinary communication and cooperation, and address issues that may impact nephrology nursing practice.

This Health Policy Statement represents the ANNA viewpoint on major public policy issues relevant to the treatment of people with kidney disease and the practice of professional nephrology nursing. This document serves to give ANNA direction as legislative and regulatory issues are addressed on local, state, and national levels. This document has been developed based on a comprehensive review of current issues and with input from ANNA members and leaders.

NURSING

1. ANNA is committed to assuring and protecting access to professional nursing care delivered by highly educated, well-trained, and experienced registered nurses for people with kidney disease.

2. ANNA supports the promotion of the registered nurse's role in health policy advocacy through educational efforts, grassroots outreach, and other activities that seek to promote the health and well-being of individuals, families, and communities affected by real or potential kidney disease.

3. ANNA supports the inclusion of registered nurses in policy development at all levels of government and on all boards, commissions, expert panels, task forces and other groups setting policies and standards that affect nursing practice, the Medicare End Stage Renal Disease (ESRD) program, and its beneficiaries.

4. ANNA supports efforts to resolve the nursing shortage, including measures to assure appropriate funding to address the shortage of nursing faculty and the availability of nursing mentors for new graduates and nurses with little practice experience.

5. Congruent with the Centers for Medicare and Medicaid Services (CMS) Conditions for Coverage, ANNA believes that registered nurses experienced in dialytic therapy must be present to provide assessment and direct supervision of patient care activities and unlicensed personnel during dialysis treatments.

Download this position statement from
https://www.annanurse.org/advocacy/resources-and-tools/position-statements

Appendix D ANNA Health Policy Statement (page 2 of 6)

Health Policy Statement
Page 2

6. ANNA believes that a registered nurse must be actively involved in determining staffing requirements in facilities providing care to people with kidney disease, and that these requirements should include consideration of patient condition and specific medical and/or psychosocial needs.

7. ANNA believes that the care of people with kidney disease is provided effectively and responsibly by registered nurses and unlicensed assistive personnel in ratios that are based on patient needs and acuity. Further, the use of advanced practice registered nurses (APRNs) in the management of people with kidney disease can result in cost-efficient high quality care, benefiting the health care delivery system in general, and the Medicare ESRD program in particular. ANNA supports the recognition of compensation for APRNs by both public and private payers.

8. Congruent with the *Medicare Improvements for Patients and Providers Act of 2008* (P.L. 110–275), ANNA believes that a sound education program is necessary to develop, maintain, and augment clinical and technical competence. ANNA believes that all licensed patient care personnel must complete a standardized nephrology education program reflecting the ANNA *Nephrology Nursing Scope and Standards of Practice.*

9. ANNA endorses the certification of qualified nephrology nurses as defined by the Nephrology Nursing Certification Commission and continuing certification to refine the knowledge of nurses providing care to individuals in all stages and types of kidney disease across the life span.

10. ANNA supports a nurse's right to refuse to perform an act or take an assignment that in the nurse's judgment is not safe or is not within that nurse's skill, experience, qualifications or capability.

11. In accordance with our commitment to compassionate end-of-life care, ANNA believes that nurses should not participate in assisted suicide or active euthanasia and that such acts are in direct violation of the American Nurses Association (ANA) Code for Nurses with Interpretive Statements and the ethical traditions of the profession (ANA, 2015). ANNA supports the ANA statement which asserts that, "Nurses actively participate in assessing and assuring the responsible and appropriate use of interventions in order to minimize unwarranted or unwanted treatment and patient suffering. The acceptability and importance of carefully considered decisions regarding resuscitation status, withholding and withdrawing life-sustaining therapies, forgoing medically provided nutrition and hydration, aggressive pain and symptom management and advance directives are increasingly evident. The nurse should provide interventions to relieve pain and symptom management in the dying patient even when those interventions entail risks of hastening death. However, nurses may not act with the sole intent of ending a patient's life, even though such action may be motivated by compassion, respect for patient autonomy and quality of life considerations."

12. ANNA believes that nephrology nurses should continue to advocate for policies and programs that promote and ensure health care environments that provide humane and dignified patient-centered care. ANNA supports continued dialogue, education, and research on end-of-life issues and appropriate decision-making related to discontinuation of or withdrawal from dialysis treatment. ANNA has commended the *Clinical Practice Guideline on Shared Decision-Making in the Appropriate Initiation and Withdrawal from Dialysis* (2010), published by the Renal Physicians Association and the American Society of Nephrology.

Appendix D ANNA Health Policy Statement (page 3 of 6)

13. ANNA believes health care personnel must be protected from occupational and environmental health hazards related to dialytic therapy and that standards for safety and protective measures should be developed, identified, and implemented.

14. ANNA believes that any efforts to detect or test for substance abuse or communicable diseases must be consistent with good medical practice and shall not violate the individual's civil rights.

15. ANNA supports the efforts of the National Council of State Boards of Nursing to implement multistate licensure for health professionals through expansion of the interstate compact.

16. ANNA supports improved provision of and access to telehealth services, both distance learning for professionals and patients as well as treatment and home monitoring of patients with chronic diseases for Medicare and Medicaid beneficiaries. ANNA supports not only the concept of telehealth but also the development of methods to reimburse providers in rural or underserved areas for these services.

17. ANNA endorses the Nursing Organizations Alliance (NOA) "Principles and Elements of a Healthful Practice/Work Environment" (July 2005), the American Association of Critical Care Nurses (AACN) "Standards for Establishing and Sustaining Healthy Work Environments" (2005) and ANA "Safe Patient Handling and Mobility: Interprofessional Nursing Standards" (2013).

18. ANNA concurs with the recommendations articulated in the report published by the Institute of Medicine titled, "The Future of Nursing: Leading Change, Advancing Health" (October, 2010). Specifically, ANNA agrees that:
    a. Nurses should practice to the full extent of their education and training.
    b. Nurses should achieve higher levels of education and training through an improved educational system that promotes seamless academic progression.
    c. Nurses should be full partners, with physicians and other healthcare professionals, in redesigning health care in the United States.
    d. Effective workforce planning and policymaking require better data collection and an improved information infrastructure.

ELEMENTS OF CARE

1. ANNA believes the practice of nephrology nursing is directed toward assessing and treating the health needs of individuals and their families who are experiencing the real or threatened impact of compromised kidney function, and/or acute or chronic kidney disease. This practice includes a commitment to help each individual and his/her significant others achieve an optimal level of functioning. Toward this end, nephrology nurses must establish high standards of patient care that are routinely updated.

2. ANNA believes that appropriate, quality treatment must be available to all individuals with kidney disease and other disease processes that require replacement therapies. ANNA supports providing these individuals with complete and accurate information about all alternative forms of therapy, including the associated risks and benefits, without regard for their cost. ANNA believes that these individuals and their significant others must be encouraged and allowed to be active participants in this decision-making process.

Appendix D ANNA Health Policy Statement (page 4 of 6)

Health Policy Statement
Page 4

3. ANNA supports legislative, regulatory, and programmatic efforts that promote prevention and management of chronic kidney disease, including early diagnosis, education and proactive creation of native fistulae for dialysis. ANNA is fully committed to working with Congress, CMS, and the larger kidney community on these issues. ANNA supports nephrology nursing participation in state and federal level initiatives to increase the use of AV fistula as vascular access for hemodialysis.

4. In order to achieve the goal of optimal rehabilitation, ANNA believes individuals must assume as much responsibility for their overall care as their physical and mental status allows. ANNA supports all home and self-dialysis modalities, with training and supervision of persons choosing these modalities being under the direction of a qualified registered nephrology nurse. Additionally, ANNA supports research into barriers to home dialysis and access to balanced education for people with kidney disease that includes home therapy as a treatment option.

5. ANNA endorses the ESRD Prospective Payment System (PPS) as established under the Medicare Improvements for Patients and Providers Act (MIPPA) and subsequent regulation from CMS and will continue to play an active role in the implementation of these changes. ANNA supports any efforts to allow flexibility for the provision of daily or more frequent dialysis, and any other safe and effective emerging treatment modalities for chronic kidney disease, including incentives for patient self-management.

6. ANNA believes that all individuals, including health care providers, must be protected from the possible threat of communicable diseases related to dialysis, transplantation, and other extracorporeal therapies and that access to testing for such diseases should be available to all patients and health care providers. ANNA endorses the vaccination of all patients against Hepatitis B, pneumonia, and influenza and the Centers for Disease Control and Prevention (CDC) vaccination recommendations for nephrology staff.

7. ANNA supports legislative, regulatory, and programmatic efforts that promote disaster preparedness and early identification, triage, and evacuation if necessary, of patients requiring kidney replacement therapy during disaster situations.

8. As stated in ANNA's September 24, 2010 letter to CMS regarding the Medicare ESRD Quality Incentive Program (QIP), as the health professional responsible for providing the majority of hands-on care for individuals with ESRD, ANNA believes that a successful and comprehensive quality incentive program must recognize the value of the nurse/patient relationship. As stated in ANNA's August 30, 2013 letter to CMS regarding the Medicare ESRD QIP, ANNA encourages CMS to consider nurse-sensitive outcome measures.

TRANSPLANTATION

1. ANNA supports public and private sector efforts to promote organ donation and increase transplantation. ANNA believes this can be accomplished by:

   a. Continued support for educational programs for the public and for health professionals addressing the shortage of donor organs and the appropriate identification of potential donors;
   b. Continued support for the federally funded Organ Procurement and Transplantation Network (OPTN) and the Scientific Registry of Transplant Recipients (SRTR);
   c. Implementation of uniform state laws regarding organ donation, procurement, and transplantation:

Appendix D ANNA Health Policy Statement (page 5 of 6)

i. Amend the Anatomical Gift Act to support that a desire to donate or not to donate expressed in any form (a donor card, driver's license check-off, placement of name on a registry, or verbal statement) cannot be revoked by the next of kin. (Indication of a desire to not donate would prohibit approaching families when there is clear evidence that the individual did not want to donate);
ii. Amend the Anatomical Gift Act to facilitate Medical Examiner/Coroner consent for 'John Doe' donations following a diligent search for identification and legal next of kin;
iii. Include organ/tissue donation language in all legislative and regulatory proposals related to advance directives, living wills, and durable powers of attorney; and
iv. Support of state registries for persons wishing to donate organs at the time of their death and federal funding for these registries.

d. Continued federal support of transplant activities including medical research and coverage of immunosuppressive drug therapy and legislative initiatives to extend immunosuppressive drug coverage for the life of the transplanted organ(s);
e. Educate insurers and other payers regarding the success and cost effectiveness of organ transplantation for their members and encourage activities that decrease actual or perceived barriers to transplantation;
f. Removal of financial disincentives to live organ donation including funding for transportation and lost income;
g. Studies to review the ethical implications of proposals to increase living non-related donation that may disproportionately affect certain populations; and
h. Support for research into the use of financial incentives for deceased donors as a potential mechanism to increase organ donation.

2. ANNA opposes coercive behavior in the solicitation of organs for transplantation and live donation when the donor's decision is based primarily on financial gain.

3. As stated in ANNA's letter to the United Network for Organ Sharing (UNOS) dated December 12, 2012, ANNA endorsed changes to the national kidney allocation system to enhance graft survival, increase utilization of donated kidneys, and improve access to kidneys for biologically disadvantaged candidates.

MEDICARE ESRD PROGRAM MANAGEMENT

1. ANNA supports ESRD payment reforms that support delivery of care and are consistent with both the standards of professional nephrology nursing established by ANNA and current professionally accepted clinical practice guidelines and standards established by the renal professional community.

2. ANNA believes that patients with CKD should have access to education, support services, and clinical care that may improve their kidney function, delay the progression of their disease, or improve their health status and readiness for the initiation of ESRD therapies.

3. ANNA supports amending Title XIX of the Social Security Act (Medicaid) to include dialysis as a mandatory service in state Medicaid programs.

4. ANNA believes that oversight of ESRD facilities should be an ongoing, collaborative effort between CMS and its contractors, including state agencies and ESRD Network

Appendix D ANNA Health Policy Statement (page 6 of 6)

organizations. Members of the on-site survey teams should be knowledgeable about the various aspects of the delivery of care to individuals with kidney disease.

5. ANNA supports the timely inspection and approval of ESRD facilities that will increase patient's access to care.

MANAGED CARE AND COMMERCIAL HEALTH PLANS AND THE ESRD POPULATION

ANNA believes that all health plans must:

1. Develop a process to ensure access to relevant specialists of members diagnosed with CKD or ESRD.
2. Develop a protocol or incentives for encouraging screening members for kidney disease and early referral of those members to nephrologists for evaluation and interventions.
3. Have a mechanism for providing access for members with ESRD to dialysis and transplant providers that are geographically accessible, whose outcomes and waiting times are known to meet acceptable national standards and averages, and that are able to provide all forms of dialytic therapy currently available, including peritoneal dialysis, home dialysis, and a dialysis schedule that conforms with the members' employment or other rehabilitation needs.
4. Involve nephrology professionals and/or utilize available clinical practice guidelines in the development of care delivery models for members with CKD.
5. Provide case management services that collaborate with nephrology providers for a comprehensive, patient centered plan of care that provides optimal kidney replacement therapy and palliative care when necessary.
6. Develop mechanisms to ensure the inclusion of members with ESRD in the ESRD Network programs and the United States Renal Data System (USRDS) database.
7. Conduct periodic evaluations of all contractors (e.g. dialysis facilities and transplant programs) providing care to members with ESRD.
8. Provide coverage for dialysis services for members who travel outside the health plan's normal coverage area.
9. Provide coverage for immunosuppressive agents for all transplant recipients for the life of the transplanted organ(s).
10. Provide coverage for hospice care.
11. Not discriminate against any policy holder in any way on the basis of a diagnosis of ESRD or condition that leads to CKD.

Adopted by the ANNA Board of Directors in March 1997
Revised and/or reaffirmed annually from 1998-2015
Most recently revised: February 2016

The Health Policy Statement is reviewed and reaffirmed annually.

Appendix E
Principles and Elements of a Healthful Practice/Work Environment

The Nursing Organizations Alliance believes that a healthful practice/work environment is supported by the presence of the following elements:

1. Collaborative Practice Culture
   Respectful collegial communication & behavior
   Team orientation
   Presence of trust
   Respect for diversity
2. Communication Rich Culture
   Clear and respectful
   Open and trusting
3. A Culture of Accountability
   Role expectations are clearly defined
   Everyone is accountable
4. The Presence of Adequate Numbers of Qualified Nurses
   Ability to provide quality care to meet client/patient's needs
   Work/home life balance
5. The Presence of Expert, Competent, Credible, Visible Leadership
   Serve as an advocate for nursing practice
   Support shared decision making
   Allocate resources to support nursing
6. Shared Decision Making at All Levels
   Nurses participate in system, organizational, and process decisions
   Formal structure exists to support shared decision making
   Nurses have control over their practice
7. The Encouragement of Professional Practice & Continued Growth/Development
   Continuing education/certification is supported/encouraged
   Participation in professional association encouraged
   An information rich environment is supported
8. Recognition of the Value of Nursing's Contribution
   Reward and pay for performance
   Career mobility and expansion
9. Recognition by Nurses for Their Meaningful Contribution to Practice

These nine elements will be fostered and promoted, as best fits, into the work of individual member organizations of the Alliance.

American Organization of Nurse Executives ~ 2004

Download this ANNA endorsement from
https://www.annanurse.org/advocacy/resources-and-tools/position-statements